EVERY BODY HURTS

Dr Chris Barnsdale

ISBN 978-1-7388700-2-8 Hardcover
ISBN 978-1-7388700-1-1 Paperback
ISBN 978-1-7388700-0-4 eBook

Media Contacts:
https://everybodyhurts.ca/
https://www.facebook.com/body.hurts/
https://www.instagram.com/body.hurts/
https://twitter.com/bodyhurt

The information presented is the author's opinion and does not constitute personalized health or medical advice. The content of this book is for informational purposes only and although the knowledge should help, it is not intended to diagnose, treat, cure, or prevent any condition or disease.

Please seek advice from your health care provider for your personal health concerns and feel free to discuss the information and health care advice from this book.

This book is dedicated to my adorable wife, Joy.
I am blessed by her love, wisdom, friendship,
and guidance every day.

Short Author Bio

Chris Barnsdale is a sports medicine doctor and author based in Alberta, Canada. Originally from England and raised on a busy dairy farm, Chris has a penchant for working hard and fixing machines. His slightly deficient brain makes him a very slow reader and causes difficulty when it comes to linear thoughts and writing words on a page.

Despite this challenge, he did well at school and started his medical education with research at Cambridge University. He flirted with surgical training, then became a GP (general practitioner), worked the ER, and finally settled in sports medicine. By focusing on understanding medical concepts rather than simply memorizing things, he has developed a unique perspective on how our bodies work and answered a lot of the questions that puzzled him and his colleagues. This book was decades in the making, as Chris sought to answer simple but tricky questions about injury, pain, healing, and body principles, and present them in a way that is easy to understand for everybody with a body.

Contents

PART 1
YOUR BODY'S CORE PRINCIPLES

PART 2
HOW YOUR BODY CHANGES

PART 3
UNDERSTANDING PAIN

PART 4
THE CAPACITY GAME

PART 5
MAKING A CHANGE

Every Body Hurts

A PHYSICIAN'S GUIDE TO
MAKING THE MOST OF YOURS

EVEN DOCTORS TELL STORIES

Hi, I'm Dr. Chris Barnsdale, the author of this book. Perhaps the most interesting fact about me is that I have the reading speed of a ten-year-old and can't write for toffee. I never felt the need to get a formal diagnosis, but my condition sometimes got in the way – I've left many exam questions blank because I couldn't read the material fast enough – but, I never let my struggles to read and write hold me back.

Luckily for me, the medical world is full of lazy examiners who prefer short answer or multiple-choice tests to long form, so I excelled in it. I even found a way to work around my condition while writing this book, by hiring a professional to help me compile my thoughts, half-written stories, and concepts. Thank you, Brittany.

Before I was a doctor, I was a dairy farmer's kid. My family had a big farm in England with 350 cows that had to be milked three times a day. I developed a strong work ethic and the realization that after being a dairy farmer, everything else is easy. I also had a strong mechanical mind. I loved working with machines, taking them apart to understand them, and learning through practice how to fix them.

As I grew into a lanky, quiet, and socially awkward adolescent, I took my penchant for hard work from the dairy farm into academics. I worked hard in school and my grades were high enough to get me into Cambridge University. More realistically, I'm sure I was accepted to fill their quota for kids from "normal" backgrounds. I remember telling a lot of jokes in the entrance interview. Funny stories go a long way, even with very clever people.

I initially started training to be an orthopedic surgeon, a career choice I based on work experience I had done in a hospital. I had watched an orthopedic surgeon cut someone's leg up with a power saw and the disbelief I felt made me to want to do it too. Surgery is, after all, just assault with a deadly weapon, but with permission.

After pursuing this career for five years, my wife and I had our first son. I fell in love with my family and started to resent the long hospital hours away from them. My love for orthopedics had been surpassed! What I really wanted to do was move to Alberta, Canada, a place I'd visited as part of a research study on osteoarthritis at the University of Calgary.

I enquired about and was offered a training in family medicine in Alberta. It meant leaving my mapped-out surgical career behind, but life is an adventure, and you only get one. Around this time, my parents, brothers, sister, and best friend all moved to Canada. What's more, my brother, sister-in-law, and best friend were all GPs and seemed quite happy.

We made the move, and our new adventure began. I started training as a GP and quickly encountered a problem. Orthopedic surgeons have a reputation for being very focused and not knowing much outside their field. There was a lot I didn't know.

I had happily slept through many of my medical school lectures or gone rowing instead. Now I had a lot to learn, and fast. My slightly deficient brain was still slightly deficient. I had never been great at remembering facts or names, and I had never finished reading a textbook. To get through medical school, I had drawn bubble maps and pictures, relied on study guides, and told myself stories that helped me understand concepts rather than memorize them. Now, facing the prospect of learning again, I became a storyteller once more.

General practice is what it sounds like. As a family doctor, you need to know a lot of things and because of this, it has become prescriptive. Family doctors are trained to see a certain thing, and then follow a protocol. For instance, if there is high blood pressure, give the patient pills and measure the blood pressure again.

I quickly became dissatisfied with this “cookbook” approach and started asking why we do it this way. The research told me that if I followed the protocols, my patients would live longer. Often my patients asked me why I was putting them on medications that made them feel worse. My answers, although correct, were often not very convincing to either of us.

I was also doing some emergency room work at this time and enjoyed applying real-time solutions to urgent problems. I missed orthopedics and in particular thinking about how the muscles and joints worked. I remembered that when I left both England and orthopedics behind, my bosses had said I was an idiot, and I would regret my decision. Perhaps they were right. I told them, “Don’t worry, I’m going into sports medicine.” This is an area of medicine where you look after people’s muscle and joint problems but offer solutions other than surgery, which is always considered a last resort.

My feelings of frustration in general practice coincided with a new clinic opening in Red Deer. It was an orthopedic surgical clinic, but they were looking for sports medicine doctors to offer a more holistic approach. Fantastic. I signed up, trying not to appear too keen.

Now I was back doing what I loved. Red Deer was an hour from the family farm where I had settled, so my daily commute was two hours a day. I spent the drives asking myself questions I had not had time to ask before. I pondered the questions my patients frequently asked me: Why is pain so unpredictable? Why is my body changing? Why can't I lose weight? What is osteoarthritis?

To find answers, I started to read papers, listen to podcasts, and consult medical research. I even went to my colleagues and asked them questions. The answers I received were usually dissatisfying, confusing, and full of medical and scientific jargon.

This inspired my journey to find simple answers to these simple questions. I started to think about the whole body. What is it for? How does it work? How does it heal? What is pain?

I began to formulate stories to explain how the body changes and shared them with my patients. They said the stories helped them better understand their bodies. With this success, I also started to tell the stories to the trainee doctors and my colleagues. They seemed to find the stories helpful too and asked more questions. One day, one of my patients was enthusiastically writing notes. She said, "Have you written this down? I would love to read a book about this if you would write one."

One of the secrets of success in life is knowing when to ask for help. It took me a long time to come to terms with my own incompetence. For me, I needed help to write this book (thanks again, Brittany). Here are my stories written down for you in the hope that you can learn what your body is telling you and get better!

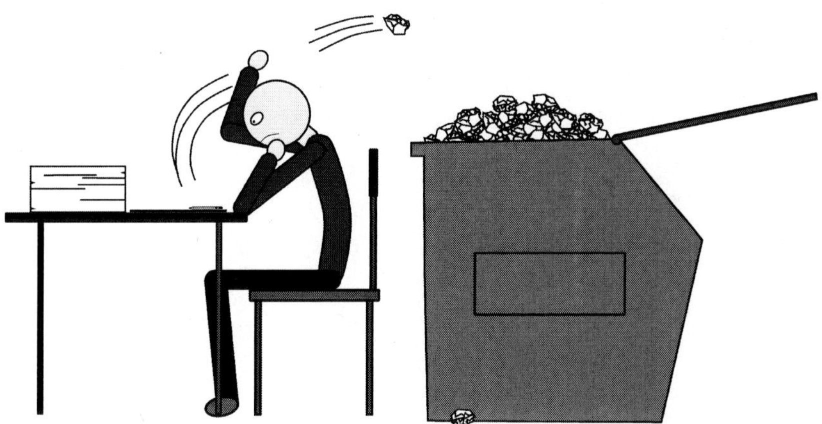

If this book looks like it was illustrated by kids, it was! Thank you to my sons Joe and Ben, for their awesome interpretations of my scribblings. Thank you also to my friend, Dean, for the couple of amazing cartoons he sketched for me. See if you can spot which ones they are!

The Purpose of This Book

I wrote this book not because doctors are lacking in knowledge or training (I promise you I'm not the smartest, most well-read doctor out there), but because while there is an abundance of experts, medical textbooks, and expanding research, there are very few simple, useful explanations on how the body works.

Most doctors can't describe in under a minute how and why your body changes. As medical professionals, we also struggle to explain why your brother hurt himself in the 5 km Fun Run while you were just fine, or why two people with an identical injury and surgery heal differently and feel different pain.

If you're reading this book, it's likely you have experienced what I call a "deconditioning event." This might be an injury that you haven't healed from. Maybe you're noticing that you are weaker and less mobile than you were five years ago. Or perhaps you're staring down at the weigh scale as the number slowly but surely goes up. Maybe you were the one who tried to do the 5 km Fun Run and limped over the finish line.

Regardless of where you are in your journey through life, I wrote this book to offer a perspective on how your body works that is based on core principles. By the end you will understand what your body does well, why you get injuries, what makes you stronger and healthier, and what factors prevent your injuries from healing.

As a curious doctor with a mechanical brain, I'm a seeker of truth and believe there are universal truths about our bodies that we simply don't know yet. Science in the modern age is still largely observational. While we make leaps and bounds in discovery, *we are still discovering things* and will be for a very long time. This means that this book may serve you, but like any other book, it is not "The Whole Truth." The truth is out there! I hope I have captured a little of it for you in here.

Here is my first story to start us off. Most people don't know how a space rocket functions in detail. If you are told to examine a space rocket and explain how everything works, you'll likely not know what the knobs and lights are for. You won't understand the wires and complex systems behind each panel you remove. However, you may be able to understand in principle how it takes off from the ground and shoots into space. You may describe pressurized gas escaping through a nozzle, causing thrust, or demonstrate the principle by blowing up a balloon and letting it go so it flies around the room.

The principle of how a space rocket works is simple. The execution of that principle is complex.

The balloon and the space rocket both use the same basic principle.
SPACE
Balloon
Rocket

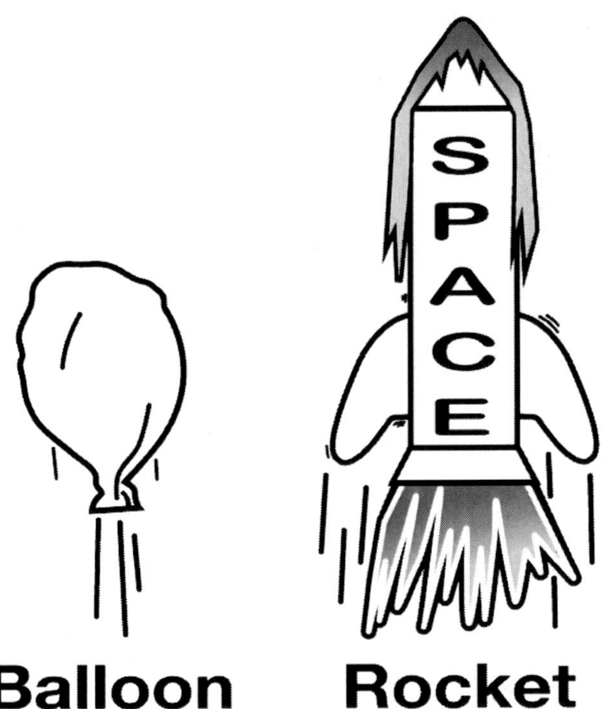

Your body is like that space rocket. In this book, you won't find unexplained medical terms or labelled anatomical drawings. Instead, this book will help you understand how your body changes, so you are better equipped to make the changes you choose to. Even more, it will teach you "body literacy": how to listen to and communicate better with your body and judge what changes are best for you.

Your body loves you; it doesn't hate you.

Although sometimes it may seem like it is actively preventing you from healing or getting stronger, in fact your body is an amazingly efficient machine whose sole purpose is to make you better. It will work to give you what you want to the best of its ability until you stop breathing. It's your job to learn how to understand your body and communicate with it, so you can *work with it, not against it*.

A Note on Sweariness

I'm not a big user of expletives (out loud, at least), but you'll find implied swearing in these pages. This is for a simple reason – this book deals with the subject of pain, which is often associated with extreme feelings. Extreme feelings make us "sweary."

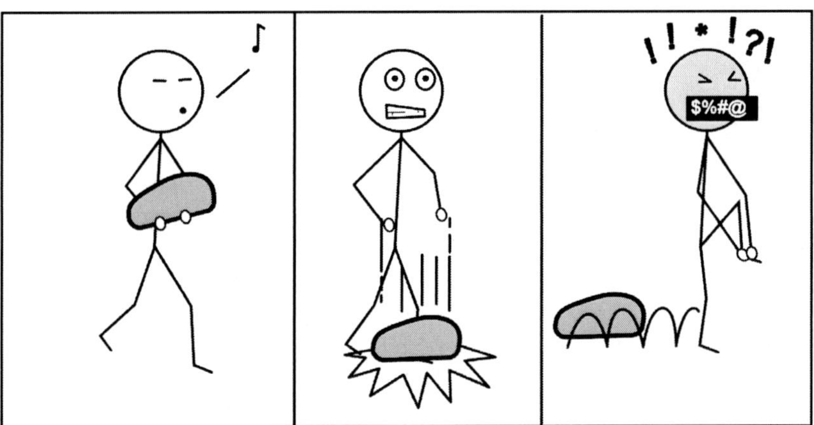

You may be a fairly benign, making-up-words, "saslafrazing nincompoopy" kind of sweary person. You may turn the air so blue that even your mother, who swears like a trooper, is disturbed by you. Medicine is full of stressed and sweary people. We often meet people on the worst day of their lives, so we get it. The implied swearing in this book is not meant to offend. Next time you drop that heavy rock on your bare foot, you'll find out if you're a sweary person too! So "shut the **** up" and read on.

PART 1

Your Body's Core Principles

Chapter 1

YOUR BODY IS A HUMAN MACHINE

As a person who loves driving, fixing, and collecting vehicles, I make a lot of comparisons between our bodies and machines. Because many of my stories are machine-based, I want to explain this principle in more detail.

Our bodies have a lot of *machine-like* qualities, but there are also ways our bodies are not like machines. The aim here is to understand your body's machine-like signals and responses as they interact with the complexity of what it means to be *human*.

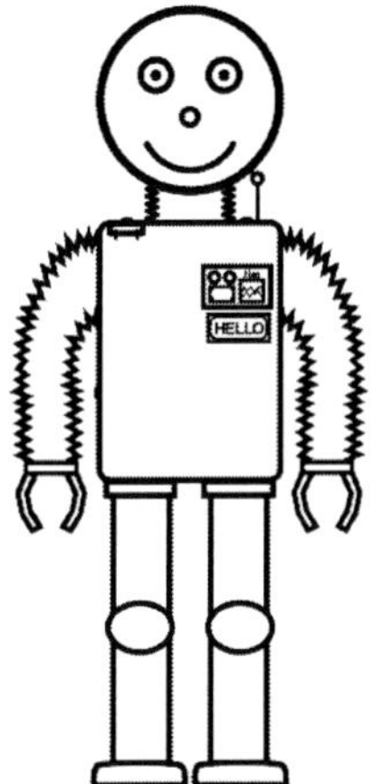

We are human machines.

Ways Your Body Is Like a Machine

1. Machines have strong similarities to other machines. Your body also has a lot of similarities to other people's bodies. We can look at a problem in one body and apply solutions that have worked for others because our systems are designed in very similar ways. This is good news! It means it's very likely that other people have experienced what you are experiencing. There are patterns and highly intelligent systems at play. You are not unknowable.

2. Machines are robust. Your body is the highest quality, most finely tuned of machines. It is designed to function well for a long time – your whole life, in fact. There are signals and mechanisms in place to respond to threats and disasters that you're not even aware of. That's how efficient your machine is.

3. A machine can communicate with the operator. Most machines let you know something is wrong with flashing lights and beeping, like when your car's "check engine" light comes on. Your body uses a similar system, only with sensations (what you feel) and emotions (how you feel). These signals provide feedback and encourage you to respond in a certain way.

4. Machines are resilient but require maintenance. Occasionally you see someone driving the same make and model as your car, but may notice that their car has rust spots, dings, scuffs, and mismatched tires. Similarly, your body is different from other people's bodies due to the decisions you make. You have the choice to keep your body in the best condition possible, or to neglect or abuse it. Like a machine, your body will do its best to keep functioning under any conditions.

Ways Your Body Is Not Like a Machine

1. Machines do not repair themselves. If you have a car crash, your car will not repair itself in the garage overnight, nor will it morph into a rally car on its own if you decide to race it next week. However, your body is intelligent, responsive, and alive. It has amazing mechanisms of self-healing, which means that you can go to sleep with sore muscles and wake up feeling recovered.

2. Machines come with a user guide. Your body does not. Some people take the time to understand how a machine works and how to care for it. For others, machines are mysteries from beginning to end. Similarly, you have a choice to get to know your body, especially as it changes and naturally wears out over time. How can you keep it strong and healthy for a lifetime.

3. You can replace a machine. Unlike a machine, your body is immensely precious. Although surgery is getting better all the time, you can't swap out your hip for a new one, like you can with brake pads, without consequences. You only get one body for your whole life.

4. Machines don't have an attitude. Your experience in your body is intrinsically affected by your beliefs. If you are convinced your car won't start, there's still a good chance it will start when you turn the key in the ignition. In other words, the car does not understand or respond to your beliefs. However, if you believe there is something wrong with your leg, you will use it differently than you would if you believed it was fine.

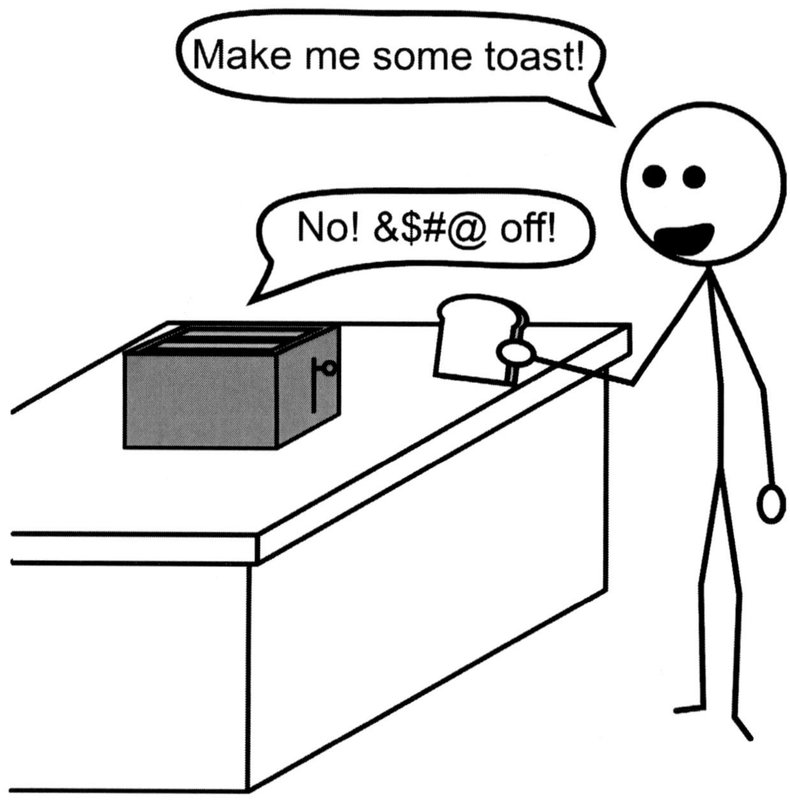

You can change the outcomes of your body by making different choices. It doesn't matter what has happened in the past or what age you are; any positive changes you begin making now can improve your body and help you live a better and longer life. This book is about how to take care of your machine to the best of your ability.

Chapter 2

YOUR BODY IS RESILIENT

Your body is meant to last a long time, and this makes it resilient. Because it responds and adapts to changes in its environment and circumstances, your body can put up with a lot of crap decisions and still function as well as it can.

Remember, your body loves you. It wants you to keep moving and living, and it has mechanisms in place to make this happen. It prioritizes what is most important to heal (things like vital organs and essential functions) over less important parts of your body. This keeps you alive and generally thriving during challenging times.

For example, if you consistently get drunk during college, your body adapts to the information you're feeding it and responds accordingly. You will find you need to drink more alcohol to feel the same effects. This may make you the envy of your friends but there will be consequences.

If you choose to train for ultra-marathons, your body will adapt to the specific strain you're putting it under. It will grow the muscles it needs to run long distances and shrink the ones it doesn't need. You will become a lean, mean, running machine.

If you break your arm and end up with a cast, the muscles in your arm will shrink from disuse while your body is fixing the bones. Once your arm is out of the cast, those muscles need to be strengthened. If you don't strengthen your weakened muscles, your body will find new, weird ways to adapt your movements, so you don't require those muscles as much.

There are consequences to any choice, although it's often hard to tell right away, because your body is good at adapting to trying conditions. It is resilient! You may not feel the consequences of binge drinking, overtraining, or neglect for many years, but they will catch up with you eventually.

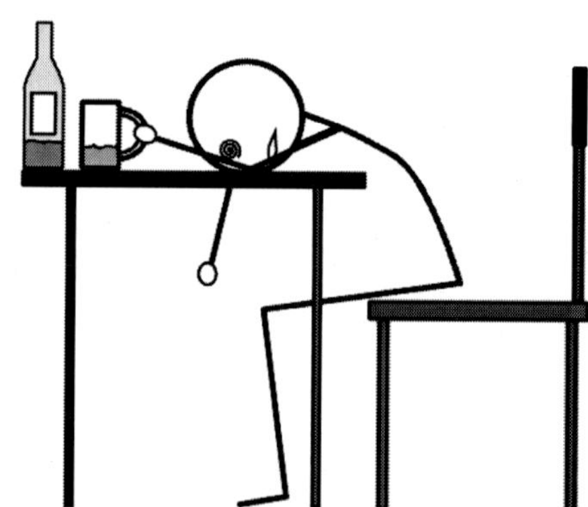

Your body is resilient and can take a lot of abuse.

Chapter 3

YOUR BODY HAS UNIQUE ADAPTATIONS

Although your body shares basic principles and mechanisms with other people's bodies, it is also a unique result of adaptations to your circumstances, challenges, and decisions. This is why no diet works for everyone, and why two different people training for the same sport in the exact same way have different results. This can feel deeply unfair.

Your adaptations come from intentional and unintentional changes that have long-term impacts. For example, say you injured your back a few years ago and have been putting up with the pain ever since. During that time, your body has developed unique adaptations that allow you to function to the best of your ability despite the injury. This means that some muscles are tighter and weaker, and some are stronger. You probably avoid certain movements that cause pain. All of this makes your body unique! Other people may just say you walk funny.

Genetics also play a role, but not always in the way we expect. Your genetics are a set of information given to you by your parents that serve as the basic building instructions for your body. I always say:

"Choose your parents carefully."

Genetics offer you the possibilities of what you *could be*. Your body has almost endless combinations of how it can assemble and adapt itself. *What you do* with your genetic information is just as important as the information itself.

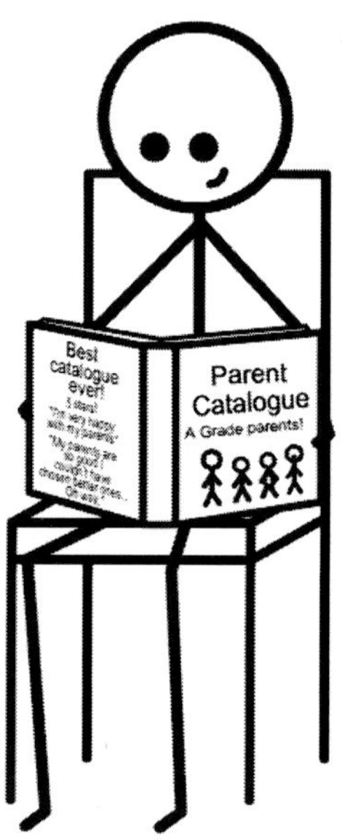

Choose your parents carefully!

As a child you grow, and your body's job is to adapt to what you do. It is constantly solving problems that you present to it by using the information in your genetic code. Your body only uses the bits of the code it needs to help you adapt to what you are asking it to do. It's important to note that some of these adaptations are not your choice. For example, what you eat as a child has a strong influence over your future eating habits. Most of us do not have much control over what we eat until we can start choosing and buying our own food.

Importantly, your body has limits to how much it can change and adapt, which are set in your genetic code. The patterns you produce from your genes during childhood are complete once you stop growing and become an adult.

Once you stop growing, what you've got is what you've got for the rest of your life.

Your unique patterns of adaptations during childhood make you an unrepeatable one-off. It is important to know that *you are much more than your genetic code*.

You may not be able to change the hand you are dealt, but you can always learn to play cards better. In other words, your job is to learn your body so well that you could write a book about it. Although your body has made these unique adaptations to try to protect you and make you better, *you always have a choice* about what to do with the cards you've been dealt.

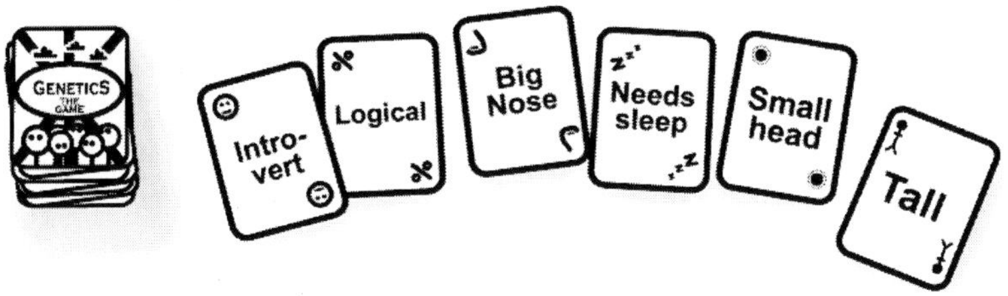

Your genes are important,
but how you use those genes is probably more important.

Chapter 4

YOUR BODY COMMUNICATES WITH YOU

The first step to making the most of your body is to understand that your body speaks to you. Just as gardeners often say their plants "talk to them and tell them what they need," your body is constantly telling you what it needs. Body literacy is the most important language that we often do not learn. In Chapter 1, I likened the body's communication system to a check engine light in a car, except in the form of sensations and emotions.

Just like seeing your check engine light flicker on, when your body sends you pain or a flood of negative emotions, it can feel more frustrating than enlightening. When you feel a stab of pain, you're more likely to think, *Ow, $#*%! than Thanks, body!*

Some people notice their check engine light come on and keep driving their vehicle until it starts to make concerning noises (this is almost always a bad idea). Others choose to look up the code associated with the light to see what's going on, and then fix the problem before it becomes a crisis. People often do the same thing with their bodies, doctors included.

If you don't understand why you're feeling an unpleasant sensation like pain, it can be an alarming and confusing experience. It's easy to believe that pain is bad when in truth, pain is simply a signal. In fact, feeling pain is a good thing and it keeps you alive. When you burn your finger on the stove, the pain you feel makes you sharply pull back, preventing you from burning your entire hand and doing irreparable damage.

Along with sensations you also feel emotions. Emotions are responses to desirable and undesirable situations. Their role is to report to you what your hormones are up to. Emotions influence how you make decisions, and this makes them very powerful. If you feel fear, you may respond by not doing whatever is causing you fear. If you feel anger, you may lash out. We will get into the relationship between emotions and the hormones that control the machinery of your body later in this book.

Once you understand that your body can communicate with you and does all the time, the next question is:

Can you communicate with your body?

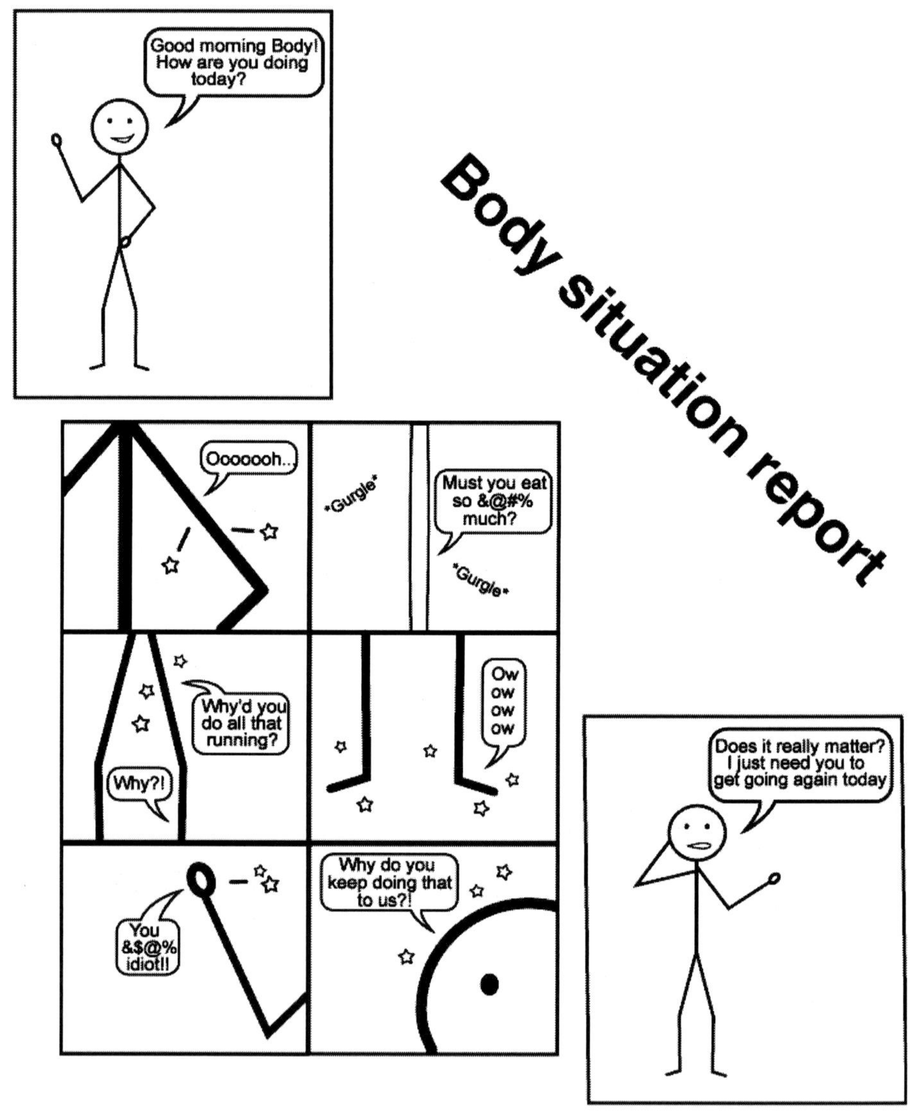
Body situation report
Good morning Body! How are you doing today?
Oooooh...
Gurgle
Must you eat so &@#% much?
Gurgle
Why'd you do all that running?
Why?!
Ow ow ow ow
You &$@% idiot!!
Why do you keep doing that to us?!
Does it really matter? I just need you to get going again today

Chapter 5

YOU CAN COMMUNICATE WITH YOUR BODY

Your body does its best to give you what you need and want. This is fantastic, but it also makes things complicated. Sometimes your goals and intentions are at odds with what your body believes is the most efficient and effective use of your resources. This is when you need to communicate with your body to let it know what you want to do and how you want it to respond.

Here is an important key:

Your body doesn't know what you want to do. It only knows what you do.

Your body speaks to you in the language of sensations and emotions, but it understands the language of action. For example, your body does not understand your intention to get stronger if you frequently sit on your couch imagining what you would look like with bigger biceps. Instead, your body receives the message to shrink your biceps because they are not being used.

If you truly want to get stronger and turn intention into results, the next step is to go to the gym and lift some weights.

Your body will listen to the input from weightlifting and respond by sending you some aching pain in your muscles and emotions like fatigue.

If you understand that your body is working on making you stronger, you will accept this potentially worrying feedback as a positive sign that your body is upgrading. Through this process, you successfully communicate with your body. By weightlifting, you let your body know what you want: bigger muscles! Your body sends you back a message, through sensations and emotions, that it's working on getting better at giving you bigger muscles! More than that, it's trying to tell you how to go about it.

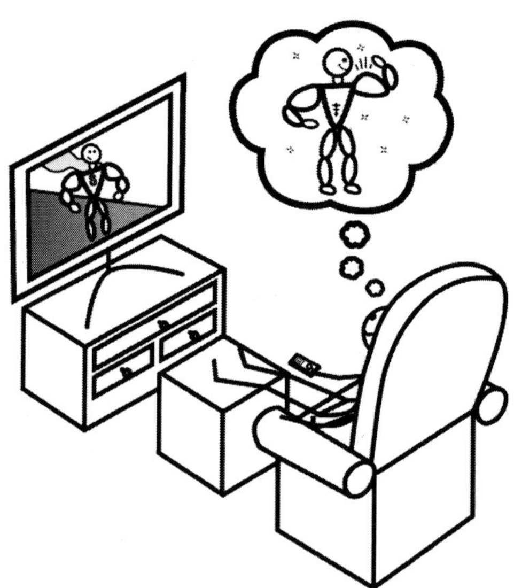

Imagining you're totally ripped doesn't make your muscles any bigger (sadly!).

Chapter 6

YOUR BODY IS ALWAYS CHANGING

Your body is always changing, whether you like it or not. There are two ways that change happens: unintentionally and intentionally. There are always results and consequences of change, no matter how that change comes about.

Unintentional change is when your body changes without purposeful effort on your part. For example, if you injure your shoulder and it stops you from doing active things you usually do, like playing baseball, your body will slowly adapt to the new conditions. This change is slow and quiet. You may not notice at all until one day when you try to swing a bat and find it awkward and painful. Another example of unintentional change is ageing. Your body naturally wears as you get older without you putting any effort into making it age. Finally, eating habits leading to unwanted weight gain is another example of unintentional change that can creep up on us.

Intentional change happens when you make purposeful efforts to change. For example, if you take the actions you need to get stronger, your muscles will grow, and your cardiovascular system will improve. You can lose weight or become fitter with intentional change.

A sneakier intentional change is when you choose to *not* do something. If I make no effort to eat well and move my body, I could frame the consequences as unintentional, but the truth is that the choice to *not* look after myself is still a choice.

Chapter 7

YOUR BODY IS EFFICIENT

You have probably figured out that intentionally changing your body can be hard to do. Why is this? It's all about efficiency. Efficiency means getting a task done with the minimum use of time and effort whilst using the smallest number of resources.

Your body has finite resources, and this is what drives its need to be efficient.

Making any physical change is a costly business for your body. When it comes to changing your body the way you want to, your body "trying to be efficient" may take some convincing to make that change. You may want to be stronger, to have bigger muscles, and to have less body fat. However, your body wants you to be very efficient, which means maintaining normal-sized muscles and fat storage so you can stay alive during any upcoming bouts of starvation. Your body is prepared for the worst.

The bottom line is that you don't need huge biceps to continue being alive, and your body knows this. Efficiency drives change, but it also makes it difficult to change when you ask your system to increase its normal capacity above what it needs to survive.

Efficiency is the body's most important operating principle.

Understanding efficiency will help you better understand how your body makes important decisions and how to make intentional changes, no matter what you have experienced. We will explore the role efficiency plays and how to work with it throughout the rest of this book.

Look after the pennies and the dollars will look after themselves.
You are so &%$# annoying.

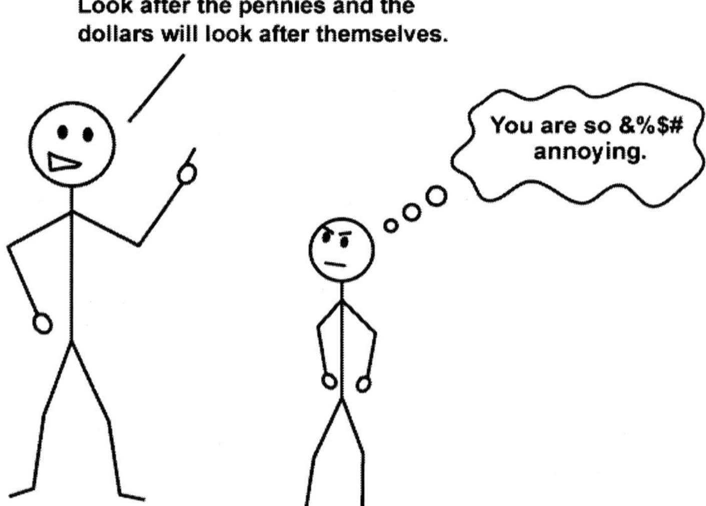

Nobody likes being told what to do!

Chapter 8

YOU ONLY HAVE ONE BODY

Your body is your most valuable investment. Yes, it is resilient, self-healing, and will put up with a lot of abuse over your lifetime, but it's not invincible. To maintain your body's strength and health, and to change it for the better, requires effort and care. Some injuries are beyond your body's capacity to heal, and there is not a second chance once this happens. You only have one body.

Making a positive change means understanding and finding the balance between experiencing some pain (which goes hand in hand with change) and overtraining, which can be damaging in the long run. Developing this awareness and knowing what to do to live a strong, long, and healthy life is what this book is all about.

The choices you make today will write the story for your body tomorrow.

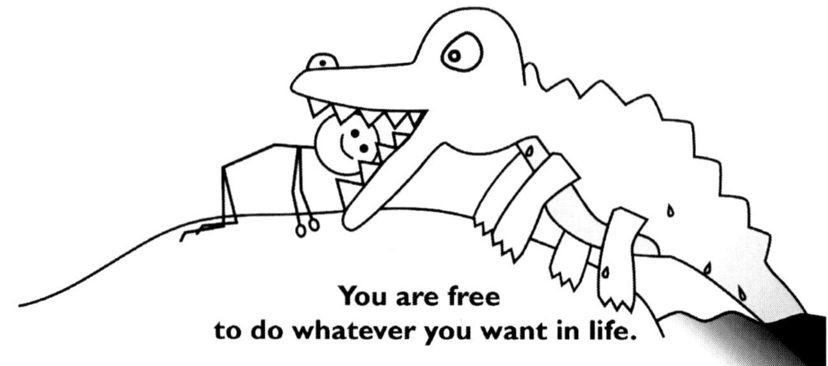

**You are free
to do whatever you want in life.**

**However, you are not free
from the consequences of your choices.**

PART 2

How Your Body Changes

Chapter 9

THE PROCESS OF CHANGE

Whether your goal for your body is to get stronger, heal from an injury or surgery, lose unwanted weight, address chronic pain, or something else, it means you are trying to create change. Learning about the process of change will help you understand why and how your body changes, what pain means, and what your body's signals are telling you.

The process of change has three steps:

1. Overload
2. Repair
3. Completed repair with upgrade

This process happens across all your systems. Your body is always assessing what needs to be prioritized and repaired.

Building Bigger Biceps

You wake up on a Tuesday morning, thinking about the hero from the action movie you watched last night. You want to build bigger biceps, starting today. What do you do next? "Go to the gym! Lift weights!" I hear you cry, and you are correct. You pull on a pair of shorts and head to the gym for the first time in years.

You know the basics of what to do at the gym; pick up a weight and lift it until you're tired. Beyond that, you don't really understand what happens when you lift weights. What makes your biceps grow? Why do they stop growing at some point? How does injury happen?

Step 1: Overload

When you walk into the gym, everyone looks like they know what they're doing. Everyone except for you. There is a helpful poster of exercises taped to a wall and you select one, a bicep curl. You look around the room for inspiration and spot a guy in the corner curling a large, heavy dumbbell. You admire his muscles.

You select a weight a little smaller than his, but still an optimistic choice considering your lack of strength. Carefully, you slide the weight off the rack with one arm. The dumbbell plunges to the floor, pulling you with it. You have just demonstrated that your arm has an upper capacity for strength and that you have exceeded it.

Looking around the room furtively, you grab the weight with both hands and haul it back onto the rack. This time, you wisely choose the smallest weight. The poster tells you to do several repetitions of the movement. It only takes a few minutes before your biceps feel fatigued and sore, so you go home, holding your freshly exercised arms limply by your side.

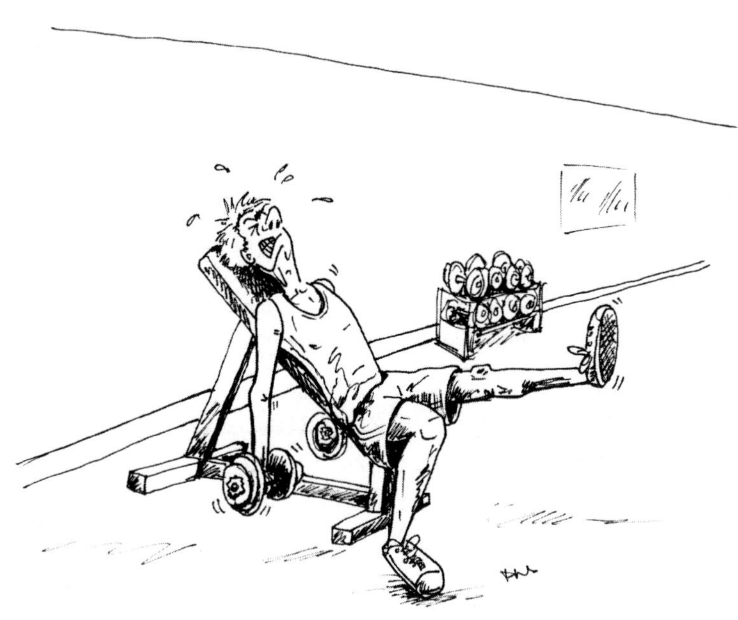

What Is Your Body's Capacity?

Aching and pain is your body's way of telling you that you have reached and exceeded your bicep's "capacity." Your musculoskeletal system (your bones, muscles, tendons, ligaments, and soft tissues) is limited and can only do a certain amount of work. In this example, you go to the gym and experience your bicep's capacity to lift a certain amount of weight. If you experiment with the weight, you will find that the heavier the weight you lift, the fewer repetitions you can do. The lighter the weight, the more repetitions. The capacity of your biceps is a combination of how heavy the weight is and how far you try to move it.

The concept of how far you can move a weight is called "work." Obviously, you can carry a pebble much further than you can move a boulder. Your capacity, the amount of work you can do, is unique to you. The guy in the corner curling a heavy dumbbell has a higher capacity in his biceps than you for several reasons, including his consistency in coming to the gym and how often he pushes the limits of his biceps' capacity.

Capacity isn't restricted to your musculoskeletal system. In fact, all your body systems have a capacity to do work. Your liver has a capacity for how much alcohol it can process before you start to feel drunk, and your lungs have a capacity for how long you can hold your breath underwater. Your body is sensitive to your needs and will do its best to adapt to any new overload it experiences. Because of this, you can expand your capacity when you cause a small overload in a system. This means doing a bit more than you can already do. When you do this, your body responds by trying to make that system stronger.

The Process of Tear and Repair

No pain, no gain!
But how the * does that work?***

"No pain, no gain" is the most common change mantra we hear but I have always been uncomfortable with this concept. Who wants to be in pain? How does hurting something make it stronger?

When you overload your bicep, you are doing some damage to it. Curling a heavy weight causes small tears in your bicep muscle. This doesn't feel pleasant, but it's crucial to push your capacity by overloading your biceps if you want to build strength in them.

Repair takes a lot of energy, which is why you can feel extremely tired when you're sick and fighting off a bug. Even a hard day at work or the gym can make you want to rest and sleep more than usual. After you get home from your first day at the gym, you start to feel a deep ache in your biceps. Although they hurt, you're happy to see that they look a little bigger than usual! As the evening wears on, they start to ache more. Eventually your arms get a bit stiff and can't straighten like they normally do. Lifting them to shampoo your hair takes more effort than usual, as does lifting a plate out of the cupboard for dinner. In fact, everything you do with your arms seems to cause you pain now. After struggling through the evening, you go to bed early and fall into a deep sleep.

Chapter 10

THE REPAIR CYCLE

The next morning dawns bright and hopeful, but your biceps feel even stiffer and sorer than they were last night. You are in the repair cycle.

Step 2: Repair

When your system is overloaded, your body's emergency services are called in to start a defend and repair program called "inflammation." This is a series of five events that is predictable and reproducible in all your body's systems:

1. Pain signals that damage has occurred from overload and tries to stop you from using your damaged body part again before it's ready. This helps to limit further damage. Pain also indicates that tissue is under repair. You instinctively treat your painful biceps carefully and avoid overloading them until they feel better.

2. Loss of function occurs in the overloaded body part. Because the area is damaged, it experiences a decrease in its capacity. This feels like weakness. In our example, lifting even a light object will be difficult when your biceps are under repair. The capacity for this part of your body slowly improves as it is repaired.

3. Swelling is used to transport emergency services to the damaged area. Your body has special cells whose job it is to repair. These "white" cells are like little repair robots. They swim in fluid, so the blood vessels become leaky around the injured tissue, allowing more of them to get to the area. The extra fluid also washes out and dilutes any contaminants and by-products produced by the hard-working emergency cells.

4. Heat in the damaged area signals that the cells are working hard. When you go for a run, you start to sweat. When you have a skin infection, it feels hot. When you get the flu, you develop a fever. This also applies to machines that generate heat. When you drive your car hard, the engine gets hot, and when you play a video game for a long time, heat is created in the gaming console. Heat indicates that extra energy is being used.

5. Redness occurs when the skin becomes flushed in its attempt to cool things down. Your body pumps fluid to the surface in lots of small blood vessels that act together as a radiator, allowing heat to escape more easily. This is why your face gets red when you run hard, and why an infected area of skin turns red.

Why Has Inflammation Got a Bad Reputation?

The moment a body part becomes inflamed, you may want to reduce it right away because it's uncomfortable. While inflammation is often seen as the bad guy, in fact the opposite is true. Think about it; we have inflammation in the world as well. When bad things happen, the defend and repair services turn up – the paramedics, doctors, fire services, police, and even the army. By inference you could say that police and paramedics are bad because they always show up when bad things happen. Of course, this is not true.

In a similar way, inflammation can also seem bad if you don't understand what it is doing. If your house was on fire, you would call fire services. Just like dousing your home in water can feel like things are getting worse before they're better, inflammation can make things harder at first. A good thing to remember is that *inflammation is not the damage itself*, but your body *limiting* damage and attempting repair. *Inflammation is the hero in the story.*

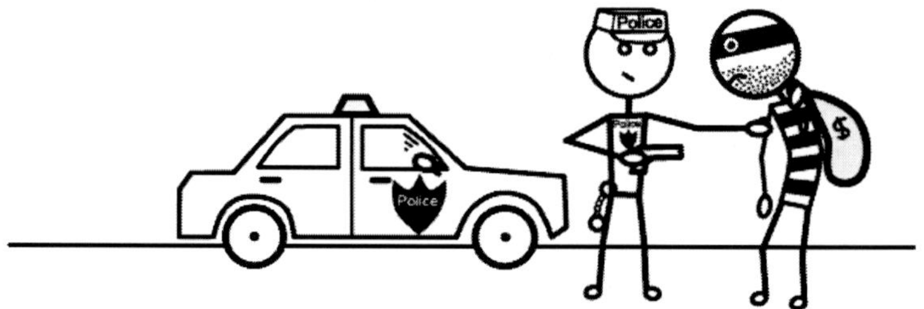

It's the Police again.
Bad things always seem to happen when they're around...

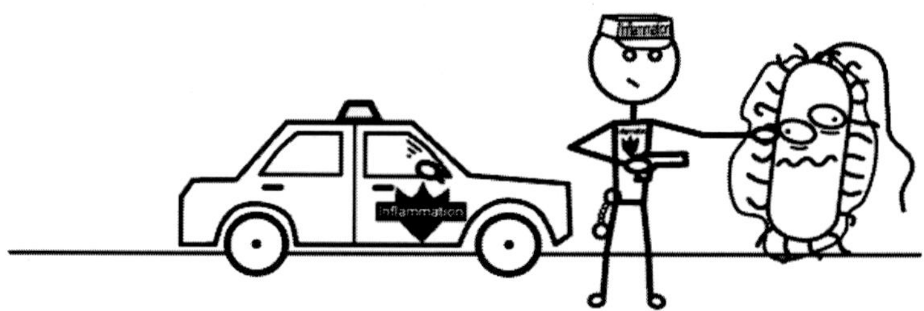

It's inflammation again.
Bad things always seem to happen when it's around...

Does This Mean Pain Is Good?

Pain can make us feel frustrated, fearful, and bad. It is uncomfortable, unwanted, always inconvenient, and can be debilitating. When you feel pain, you might think:

Oh $#*%, have I ruined my body forever? Remember that pain is a signal telling you what to do, which is to let your body repair itself to the best of its ability.

In our biceps example, the pain is telling you *not* to lift more heavy weights for a while. It's saying, "I've got this. Let your biceps heal." If you choose to push through the pain and keep lifting heavy weights with your sore biceps, you'll find that your muscles ache even more and that you have less and less capacity with each effort.

The biggest problem is that pain is ****ing painful!

I think we all prefer not to feel pain. However, it's good to remember that pain plays a key role in change, as well as your survival. It serves as a gauge for how much damage you're doing, so that you can overload and repair effectively without risking more extensive damage. The purpose of pain is to protect the injured system from further overload while it is under repair. Be thankful that you can feel pain!

Step 3: Completed Repair with Upgrade

It's been a few days since your initial trip to the gym. The aching in your biceps has subsided enough for you to consider lifting weights again. In fact, not only has the pain gone away, but your muscles feel better than ever! You feel a little stronger and when you lift the same weight as last time, it feels easier.

Your body is amazing. Not only does it repair small injuries, but it goes the extra mile and improves your system, anticipating that change will keep happening. We will talk about this upgrade process more in the following chapters. Remember, your body doesn't understand what you *want* to do, it only understands *what you do*. By causing a small overload, you are telling your body to prepare for more work of this kind in the future.

This step in the repair cycle is called "completed repair with upgrade." An upgrade can only happen when the repair cycle has completed, which means when the pain has gone (think of a traffic light signalling green). In other words, don't go back to the gym until your muscles feel recovered! Your body will try to give you the biceps you want if it is given the chance. Most prolonged pain that lasts months or even years happens because a repair cycle was *not* able to complete before the next overload happened. If you are recovering from a serious injury, or have in the past, ask yourself whether you may have caused overload in the middle of a repair cycle, preventing it from completing.

Chapter 11

GETTING A SUNBURN

Let's test the process of change with a completely different example. When you go to the gym and work hard to build bigger biceps, the change you make is generally intentional and positive. What about when the change is unintentional and negative? Does the process hold true?

The Sunburn

It is a spring weekend, and the sun is out for the first time this year. People are flocking to patios to share a beverage with their friends, including you. You dig out a sleeveless shirt from the bottom of your drawer and bath your arms in the warming sunshine. *I'll only sit in the sun for a couple of hours,* you think, hoping to get a light tan.

The warmth feels nice on your skin, and a cool breeze refreshes you. *It's not that hot,* you think. After two hours, you go home and hop in the shower. The hot water hits your arms. "$#*%!" you yell, as you feel instant, shocking pain. When you get out and look in the mirror, you discover that your exposed skin is bright red. On top of that you have some new, and very unfortunate, tan lines. Right now, they are burn lines.

Step 1: Overload

Just like your first time at the gym, you have overloaded your body's capacity. In this case, you have overloaded your skin's capacity to be in direct sunlight. After a long winter of covering your arms up, your skin's capacity under the summer rays is very low indeed. Although the sun gives your body great things, including vitamin D, which is essential, too much of a good thing can be bad.

Although it doesn't feel the same as lifting weights, your skin has done a lot of work by protecting your body from the sun's damaging UV rays. And just like the biceps example, your system is signalling damage and overload, prompting you to stay inside for the rest of the evening.

Step 2: Repair

The next morning, your skin is very tender and deeply red. Even rubbing soft fabric across it is enough to cause prickles of pain. This pain signals that your skin is under repair and encourages you to stay out of the sun or cover up to avoid more damage. The emergency services have arrived and are hard at work. You notice:

1. **Pain.** Your skin is tender to the touch.
2. **Loss** of function. You instinctively avoid rubbing your burnt skin.
3. **Swelling.** When you press lightly on your arms, your skin feels a little tight. The extra fluid in the injured area presses back against your fingers.
4. **Heat.** Your skin is radiating warmth as your cells go to work, repairing the damage.

5. Redness. Wherever the sun has caused damage, the skin now looks bright red. This is because the skin's blood vessels dilate, fill with warm red blood, and act as a radiator to help cool the body.

Once again, inflammation and pain come to your rescue. If you were to go back outside the next day and expose your burned skin to those UV rays, you would experience more pain and damage in the form of a deeper redness and maybe even blisters. Luckily for you, your body is a good communicator, and you choose to stay inside.

Step 3: Completed Repair with Upgrade

After a few days, the soreness of your burn dies down, and you don't feel the same level of swelling and heat. The redness also fades, leaving behind tanned skin, which is more resistant to the damaging effects of sunlight. Your body anticipated future change and has responded by making your skin less likely to be injured the same way again.

Just as you could lift more weight at the gym after the repair cycle completed, you can now spend more time in the sun without getting burned. Your skin has been upgraded! However, this change can have consequences. If from this point onwards you choose to spend a lot of time in the sun without protection, you may risk health complications like skin cancer.

Training your system to be stronger and more resilient isn't always a good thing when the overload is too great, or the damage is due to something that is harming your body. In this case, UV light damages the DNA inside your cells. Even repeatedly lifting weights that are very heavy or running too far regularly can be bad for you. More on this later.

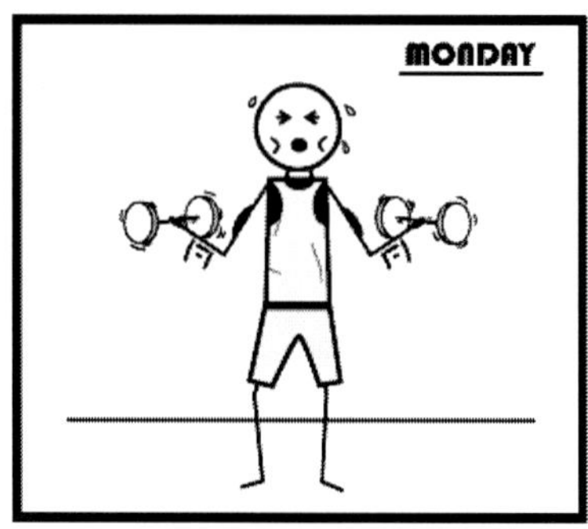

Hard

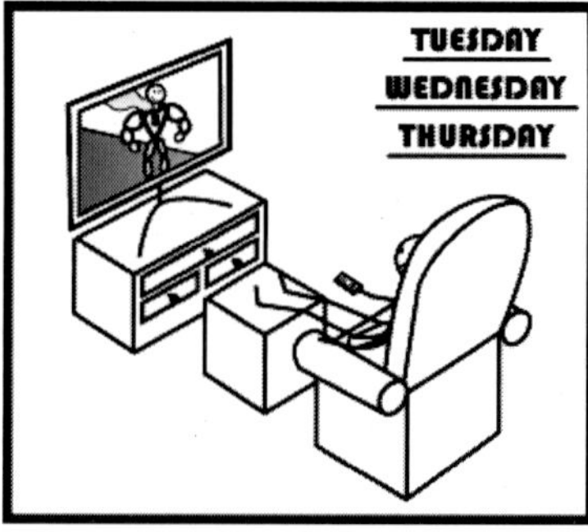

The best way to upgrade your body is full recovery.

I'm *not* being lazy.
I'm getting stronger by letting my body finish repairing.

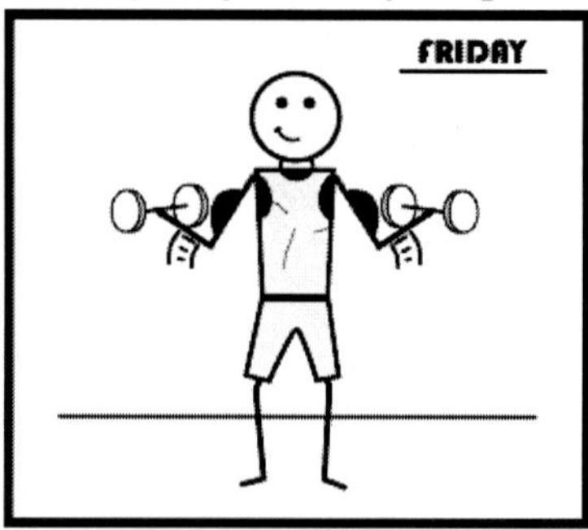

Make sure your body feels recovered and isn't aching when you go to train again.

Upgrade = Easier

*Results may be exaggerated for illustration purposes.

Two Keys to Creating Change

You have probably experienced this cycle of overload and repair. Another word for it is "training." Whether you're lifting weights or getting a sunburn, training your body is how you create change. There are two important keys to creating positive change that sticks, without causing further injury:

1. Always allow your body to complete the training cycle before overloading it again. To get the upgrade, your body must be able to finish the repair.

2. Be consistent. Repeatedly going to the gym after the repair cycle has completed helps train your muscles to grow over time. You'll notice that people who go to the gym regularly have strong, well-defined muscles.

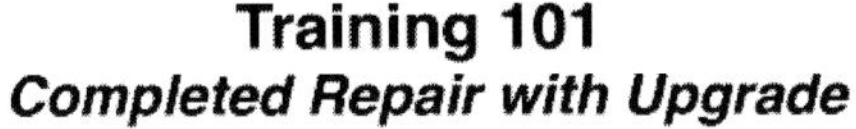

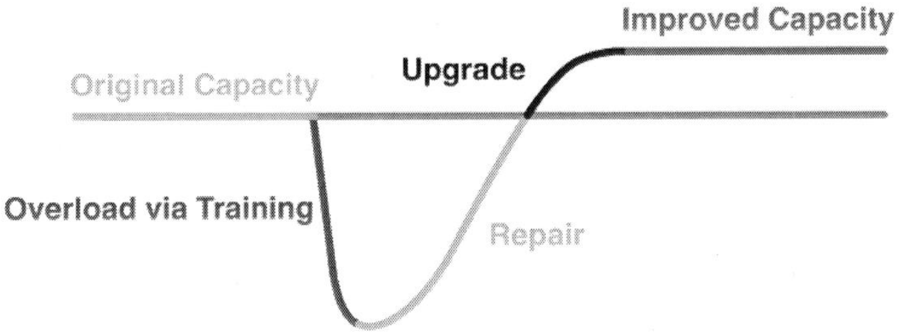

In the next chapters, we will get into the topics of capacity and efficiency to understand the impact of the overload and repair cycle over your lifetime, how your body decides what to change and how, and why some changes you make don't seem to stick.

Chapter 12

WHY YOUR CAPACITY MATTERS

Back to the gym! Let's fast forward a few weeks. After your initial brush with overloading your biceps, you have been lifting weights regularly and figuring out how to train your muscles. You stop when you feel pain (tear), allowing your muscles to recover (repair) for a day or two before going back (completed repair with upgrade). After a while you notice you can lift heavier weights and do more repetitions. You are stunned by the results so far. Your arms, once rather shapeless, are now becoming toned and strong. There's no denying it – you are on the road to looking like that hero in the action movie.

Over time you get serious about developing your muscles, and you notice that your rate of improvement is flattening. Although you are going to the gym frequently, you aren't seeing the same gains. Why is this happening? The answer lies in your capacity and the inherent efficiency of your body. Let's start with capacity.

Your whole body is limited by the number of resources it has available.

You need to use your body's stored energy and raw materials to operate its machinery. For example, to upgrade your muscles, you need to burn fuel to run the repair machinery that fixes the damage you do as you train. However, the same fuel that runs your muscles is also used to run your brain, heart, lungs, guts ... all your systems. This is where your "fitness" comes in.

I'll use the example of a turbocharger on an engine to illustrate how this works. The power of an engine depends on how much fuel it can burn. How much fuel it can burn is determined by the amount of air available to burn the fuel. To gain extra power in an engine you can add a turbocharger, which is a fan that blows air into the engine. The extra air allows the engine to burn more fuel, which means it can do more work. This increase in "power" can be used to make the vehicle go faster.

The same thing happens in your body, where the limiting factor in doing work is how much energy can be made. The capacity of your cardio-respiratory system (heart and lungs) limits how much overall work your body can do. Like an engine, how much fuel you can burn is limited by how much air you can breathe. You use oxygen to "burn" your body's fuel.

A measure of your body's cardio-respiratory capacity can also be called "how fit you are." Your fitness is essentially how much air you can breathe to supply oxygen, burn fuel, and then remove waste gases produced by burning the fuel. The maximum volume of gas you can move can be measured while you do exercise, giving you a maximum value, or VO2 max. This number is a bit like the horsepower of your car. The bigger your VO2 max, the more work you can do.

Just as a car only has so much power and can only go so fast, once you max out your available resources, you are exceeding your capacity and entering whole-body overload.

You can max out what your body can do.

You may stop seeing improvements in the gym for two reasons. The first reason is *inadequate resource intake*. This is simply not eating enough food *or* not eating enough of the right things! You need fuel in the form of food to run your machinery, and raw materials including lots of protein to rebuild and repair your muscles as they do more work and get injured. If you aren't eating enough protein, you may have reached your body's capacity to repair your torn muscles. When this happens, you will find that, try as you might, you just can't get any stronger. Muscles are made of protein!

This means that if you are aiming to lose weight *and* build bigger muscles at the same time, you can hit your repair limit quickly. The "bootcamp-style" fitness program is a common example of eating very little and exercising hard. I'll speak in more detail about bootcamps later in this book.

The second reason you may stop seeing improvements at the gym is less common: *improper training*. If you aren't seeing improvements and you are eating enough, you have either reached your potential capacity or you are not training effectively. For example, if you continue to lift around the same amount of weight the same way, week after week, the work that once exceeded your capacity becomes comfortably *within* your capacity. Overload is what tells your body to increase capacity. This means that when you stop overloading, your capacity also stops increasing. You're going to have to overload more to see more gains.

Potential Capacity

At the gym, you realize you've been lifting the same weights the same way for a long time and not making progress. You decide to invest in professional help.

Your personal trainer helps you optimize your body for building muscle. With a special training and eating plan, you start to make big gains. The changes you see in your body are now coming closer to the muscular hero that inspired you.

After a year or two of training, you start to notice that once again, you aren't really improving anymore. You have reached the limit of what your muscles can do under these conditions. You are officially "maxed out," which means that no matter how hard you train, or how much you change your diet, you won't get any stronger.

This maxed-out moment is what pushes some body builders to use steroids, which tell your body to go beyond its programmed limits. This is not a good idea. Steroid use can push upper limits of muscle capacity to the point where muscles may even tear off bones! They also damage other systems in the body. For example, long-term steroid use can increase the risk of liver cancer.

By now you know that all your body systems have an upper capacity, and you can improve your capacity through the process of overload and repair. Now you are confronting your body's *potential capacity*, or absolute upper limit. Not many people are dedicated to training enough to ever reach their potential capacity.

How Much Can You Change?

Determining the upper limit of what your body can do is complicated. There are many factors that impact your upper limit, including

1. Genetics: What information your parents gave your body to work with
2. Childhood: The lifestyle and activities you experienced as a child
3. Past injuries: Major injuries that may have permanently damaged parts of your body
4. Nutrition: How well you ate from childhood to the current day
5. Age: Once you become an adult, your body begins to slowly wear out over time. This causes your upper limit to decrease as you get older. We will talk more about this later.

Your upper limit is unique to your experiences and what you did with the genetic information your parents gave you. When you were a child, what you did affected how your body grew. During this time your body was essentially trying to guess what you were going to do when you became an adult. It did its best to adapt and prepare to be an adult based on what you did when you were still growing.

A Note on Genetics

Genetics is a huge topic, and one that I cannot do justice to in this book. However, there are some important things to consider when it comes to genetics that I will touch on. First is the tendency to lean on or blame genetics for things that go wrong in our bodies. We all get slightly faulty genetic information from our parents that can affect how our bodies are made. However, these minor faults rarely affect your body's real-world functions. No car is made perfectly either. Very occasionally, a manufacturing defect will be substantial enough to affect your car's functionality. The truth is

What you do with the genetic information your parents gave you is more important than the genetics themselves.

How you were made – the information passed to you by your parents – sets the upper limits of what you can achieve. This is a combination of the genes you were given (genetics) and what genes were used (epigenetics) through adaptations your body made while you were growing. How you customized your body during your growth phase sets your potential upper limits. These are the upper capacity limits of what each of your body's systems could reach.

This is why some of us are more natural runners, thinkers, or musicians. If we excel in these areas (in other words, we have a higher capacity to do them compared to others), it is due to a combination of our genes and what we chose to do with them. This is deeply complex.

The most important thing to understand is that as an adult, your potential capacities are set. It is entirely up to you how close to your potential you want to get. You can get closer to your potential capacity by training specific parts of your body through the process of overload and repair.

A Tale of Two Brothers

To illustrate the power of choice we have within the limitations we have, let's look at machines again, this time, the simple flywheel. The flywheel in an engine is a heavy metal disk that the engine spins. As it spins faster, the flywheel gains momentum by using some of the engine's energy. This means that the heavier the flywheel is, and the faster it spins, the more momentum "energy" it has and the harder it is to stop it spinning.

When you start a new activity you "build a habit flywheel"!

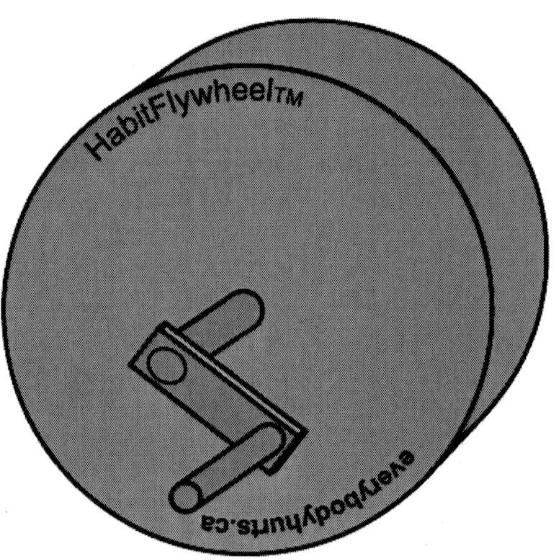

The more you do the activity the faster it spins and the heavier your flywheel gets.

You have metaphorical flywheels that represent any activity your body does, the things you do habitually. When you start to do an activity you "build" a flywheel, which takes energy and resources. The *speed* at which your "habit flywheel" spins represents how often you do that activity. Think of this as tapping the flywheel to make it spin, every time you do the activity. The flywheel's *weight* represents the quantity of the activity you do. The greater the quantity of the activity the heavier the flywheel.

This means that someone who swims three days a week will have a faster spinning flywheel than someone who swims once a month. The weight of the flywheel will be greater if they train to swim twenty lengths of the pool than if they only train to swim ten lengths. A devoted swimmer who has been swimming since the age of ten will have been tapping the "swimming flywheel" for longer than someone who only started swimming a few weeks ago and so the speed will be higher.

The combination of these two factors creates a "habit momentum." This is your capacity to do the activity. In our example, combining swimming three times a week since childhood (flywheel speed) and swimming twenty lengths of the pool (flywheel weight) would produce the greatest habit momentum. Habit momentum represents how much your body has invested in this activity and is therefore how easy it is for your body to do that activity.

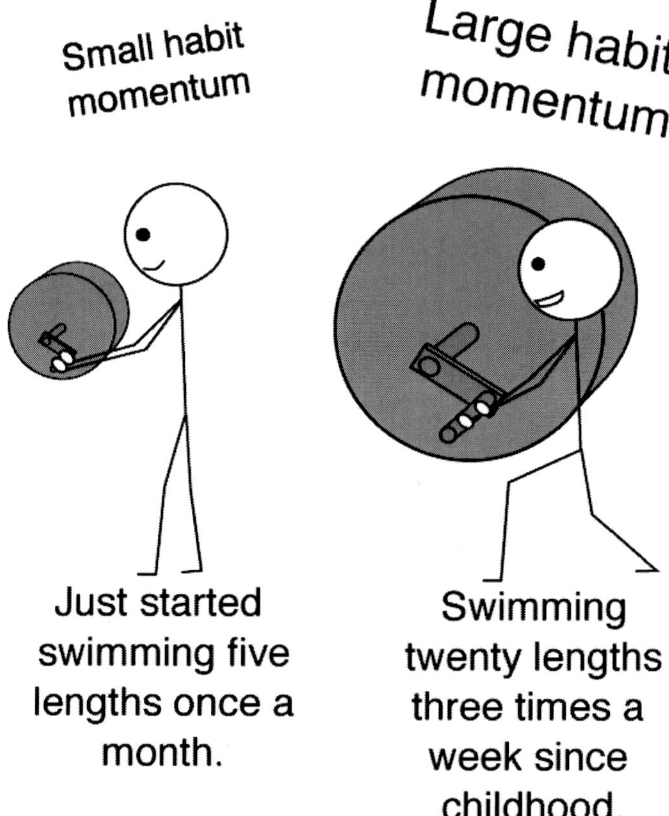

The tale of two brothers is about a pair of identical twins, which means they are genetically the same, are the same age, and had similar upbringings. One brother likes to run. He has been running 5 km two or three times a week for fifteen years. In flywheel language, his running flywheel has *quite a lot of momentum* (it has 5 km of weight and spins at fifteen years).

The second brother recently took up running. He has been training hard over the past three months to be like his brother and run 5 km. He can now run 5 km comfortably and does so two or three times a week. His running flywheel has *much less momentum* than his brother's (it has the same 5 km of weight but spins at only three months).

Let's say that both brothers decide to *stop* running on the same day. Both their running flywheels now have no input to keep them spinning so they start to spin down, which means they spin slower over time.

The first brother's flywheel has more momentum, as it is spinning faster, so it spins down less. The second brother's flywheel is spinning slower, so it loses momentum more quickly. A few months later, the second brother's flywheel is spinning much slower than his brother's.

How easy it is for each brother to run any distance depends on how much running habit momentum is retained in their flywheel. After three months of rest from running, the brothers agree to go for a run together. The first brother finds he can still comfortably run 4 km, which is his new capacity after his break. His running flywheel has only spun down by 1 km because it still has more momentum. Meanwhile, the second brother struggles to run any distance at all. His running flywheel has spun down and stopped, as if he had never trained.

This flywheel analogy can be used for other examples in your body. Your whole body has an activity momentum. When we think about potential capacity – your absolute upper limits – we are talking about your maximum flywheel momentum. Although these twins are genetically similar and grew up together, they did something different with the information given to them and experienced very different results.

For the ambitious people out there, remember that

There is only so much your whole body can do.

There is only so much you can do.

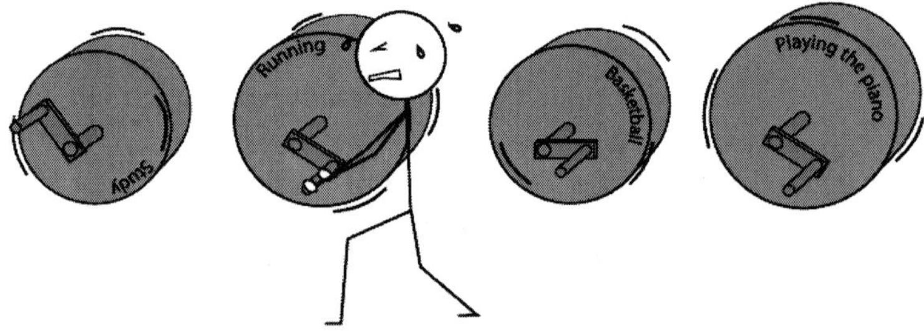

You can do multiple activities,

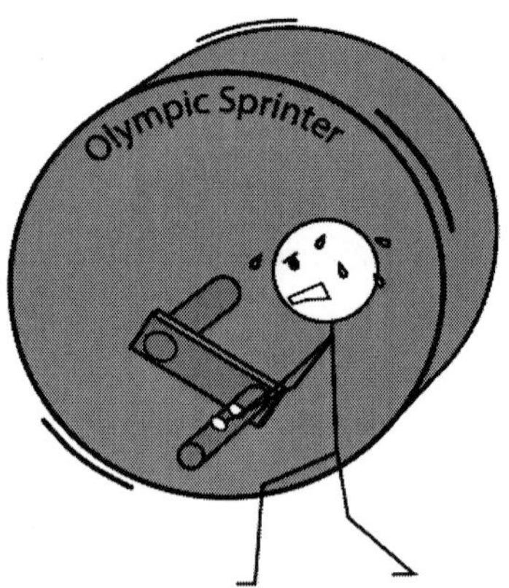

or you can specialize and put all your efforts into one activity.

You only have enough resources to build and keep so many flywheels spinning at a time. There aren't many of us who can run a four-minute mile, then whip up a perfect souffle while expertly playing a violin and brokering a million-dollar deal on a Bluetooth headset. I suspect even Clark Kent was a mediocre reporter!

Another Dog got stuck in a drain today, and the firebrigade came and pulled it out and it was safe and the owner was happy.

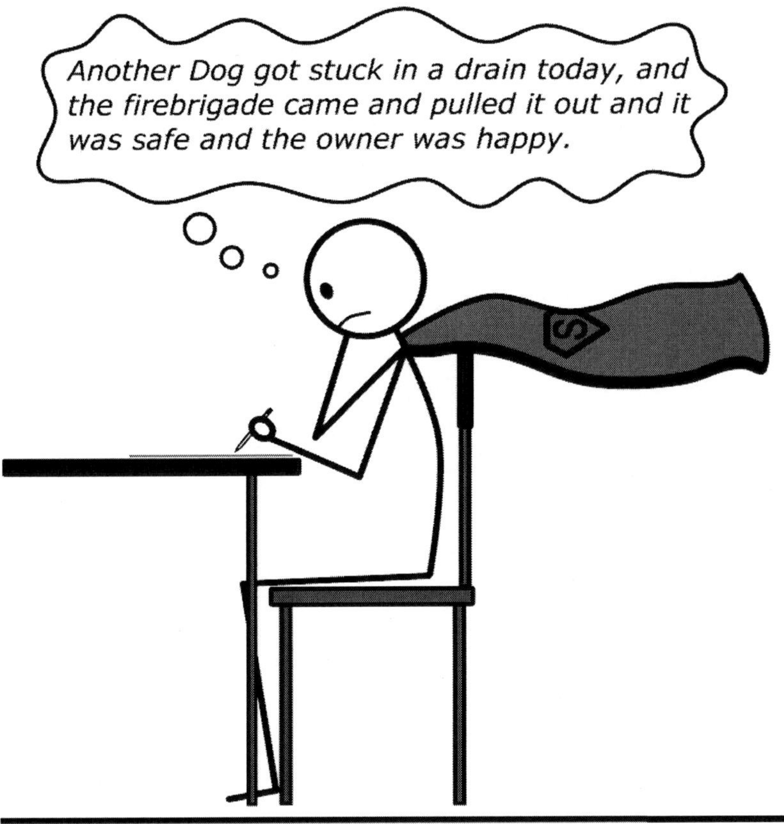

Clark Kent was probably an average journalist.

In addition to capacity, there is a second, very important aspect of your body to take into consideration as we venture further into the journey of change: efficiency. The principle of efficiency is what drives your body to change, but it can also hinder the changes you want to make.

Chapter 13

THE ROLE OF EFFICIENCY IN CHANGE

As you learned back in Chapter 7, your body is an efficient machine. Because your body has a finite number of resources at its disposal, its main job is to use those resources as efficiently and effectively as possible. There is only so much it can do in a day, so prioritizing and distributing resources is your body's main job. It is not an exaggeration to say that

Everything your body does is about efficiency.

Understanding this concept will help you understand the changes (or lack thereof) you experience in your body. Repairing an overloaded muscle is a very expensive process for your body. It requires a lot of energy and raw materials, something you feel during the process of inflammation as aching and fatigue. A lot is happening in your body to ensure that your injury is fully repaired.

If you repeat the activity that caused overload the first time, for instance by going back to the gym regularly, that muscle will be damaged again and again. Your body knows this, so to save costly resources, it chooses to upgrade the muscle to make it stronger.

It is cheaper to repair and upgrade than repair the same injury twice.

Using this upgrade process, it works hard to adapt and change in anticipation of future damage. As you learned, this upgrade is why it is easier to lift weights when you return to the gym.

Your body manages its resources like an accountant looking over a balance sheet. Since it knows repairs are expensive, your body will only upgrade something if it will save resources in the long run. If you overload a muscle, your body knows that repairing the same injury over and over again in the future will be so expensive that it makes more sense to avoid the need for future repair by investing in an upgrade now.

Your Body Is Like a Shoe Factory

From our earlier discussions on capacity, you know that if your body can meet the demands placed on it, nothing changes, which is why your muscles don't get stronger if you continue to lift the same amount of weight every day. If there is excessive demand, then your body changes to meet this demand. Now, to understand efficiency in real terms, let's consider a shoe factory.

This shoe factory has a capacity to make a certain number of shoes per day. For years, it has functioned within its capacity, until one day there is a huge rise in the demand for shoes. To meet the demand, the factory must increase its production. The simplest way to do this is to run the production line machinery as quickly as possible. Everything in the shoe factory gets a lot faster and noisier. Eventually, the machinery hits its upper limit and cannot go faster – but the demand keeps rising. Now there is a real danger, because the machinery is running slightly above its safety capacity, getting hot, and making concerning sounds. If it runs at this level for too long, it will eventually break down.

The shoe factory manager makes a wise decision. Once the order is completed, he calls for the production line to be repaired and upgraded. He anticipates that there will continue to be a high demand for shoes, so while the current machinery is being repaired, he orders more machinery to be installed. He knows two things: First, that it's more efficient to increase the capacity of the factory than to have to repair the machinery again in the future. Second, he knows that repairing and upgrading the machinery will take some time. As a result, the factory is partially shut down while the repairs are made. It runs at a reduced capacity, and customers are told that they may have to wait longer for their order to be filled.

Once the repairs and upgrades are done, the shoe production line is ready to make more shoes. It can handle larger orders comfortably within its new capacity, and now the machines are much less likely to be overworked and require additional expensive repairs. It is important to complete these repairs and upgrades before running the production line again, because opening the factory too soon or rushing the repairs could cause more trouble.

A few months later, the fashion trends shift and the demand for these shoes drops off. The factory now has the opposite problem – there is excessive capacity in the shoe production line. Some machines aren't even being used anymore. It is inefficient and expensive to keep running all this machinery for so few shoes.

The savvy factory manager now has a tough decision to make; he tries to judge how long it's worth keeping the expanded production lines open. If the demand has been strong for years, he is more likely to keep extra production lines open, assuming the demand will return to normal in due time. If demand stays low for a long time, or it was only high for a short period, he orders the extra machines to be turned off. After a few more months of decreased demand, the factory manager decides to sell unused machinery because otherwise they would require monthly maintenance costs and use of resources.

Efficiency Is the Driving Force behind Repair Upgrade

Your body's systems behave the same way as a shoe factory. If your body experiences excessive demand on a system, as demonstrated by going to the gym for the first time, overload happens. Because your body is efficient, the system is also upgraded to avoid the expense of repairing a repeated injury in the future.

If you stop going to the gym, there is suddenly an excess of capacity in the system. For you, it means that when you stop lifting weights, your biceps are now stronger than they need to be to carry out everyday tasks. Just like the shoe factory, your muscles will be "turned off," shrinking and weakening over time to avoid using precious energy to maintain something that isn't being used.

Your body is responsive and loves you. It wants you to thrive. However, even if you want your bigger biceps to stick around, you are telling your body to stop spending energy on them when you stop using them.

Status: normal
On
On
On
Status: low speed
On
Off
On
It's easy to turn things off or turn things down
Status: OVERDRIVE
ON
ON
ON
Running over capacity is hard on the machinery
Status: upgrade
Off
Off
Off
It's slower in the short term but more efficient in the long term to upgrade things
Machine Parts
Machine Parts
Egz

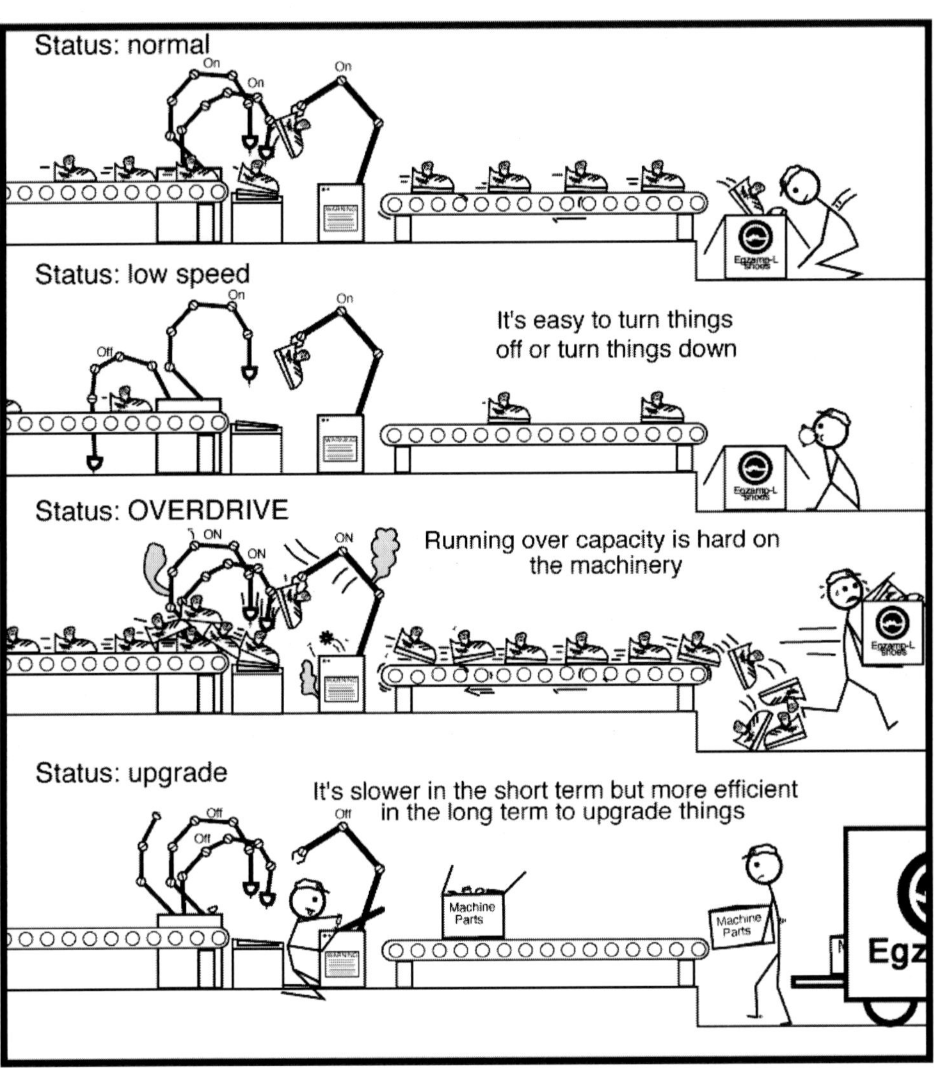

Managing a shoe factory

Remember, your body doesn't understand what you *want* to do, only *what you do*. In fact, your body is helping you thrive by re-allocating those precious resources to other parts of your body.

Because of efficiency, your body turns things off quickly to save resources but invests slowly in expensive upgrades. Essentially, efficiency is the reason you experience an upgrade like stronger muscles, and it's also the reason your body saves resources for the future, which is why you can put on unwanted weight. We will talk more about this in Part 4.

But before we go there, let's explore what happens when your body simply cannot repair – when you inflict an injury beyond the capacity of your body to heal on its own. What happens when there is too much overload?

Chapter 14

WHEN YOUR BODY CANNOT FULLY REPAIR

To upgrade and improve your body, the process of change (overload, repair, and completed repair with upgrade) is necessary. You learned that your body is very efficient, and that efficiency is the driver of repairing and upgrading the small injuries you cause during overload, to avoid more expensive repairs in the future.

Sometimes your body cannot complete the repair cycle. If you go back to the gym too soon, before the repair and upgrade process is complete, your muscles will tear even more, causing more inflammation. If you head out into the sun the next day after getting a sunburn, your sunburn will get worse. We call this repetitive strain "overtraining." Even if your intention is to grow bigger muscles or to develop a nice tan by pushing your capacity, your body (say it with me), doesn't understand *what you want to do*, it only understands *what you do*. When you insist on pushing your capacity before the repair process is complete, what your body understands is that repetitive injury is the new norm.

Here are a few examples of system overload we can all recognize:

1. Abdominal pain from eating too much

2. Burning your hand on a stove
3. Breaking a bone from a fall
4. Getting a hangover from drinking too much alcohol
5. Hitting your thumb with a hammer

For all these examples, there is a balance between the amount of damage that happens and the amount of repair that can be done.

Keeping this balance on the side of repair is very important.

For change to be successful, your body needs to be healing more than it is getting hurt. Burning your hand on a stove can be repaired. Repeatedly burning your hand becomes a problem. Breaking your leg means that you're in for a lengthy repair but taking your cast off too early can have catastrophic, long-term effects.

Some injuries are so big, our bodies cannot fix them. For example, breaking your neck and severing your spinal cord or chopping off your leg are irreversible injuries. In the most dramatic examples of overload, it is possible to suffer an injury that is big enough to overload the whole body and cause "total body failure," which is also known as death.

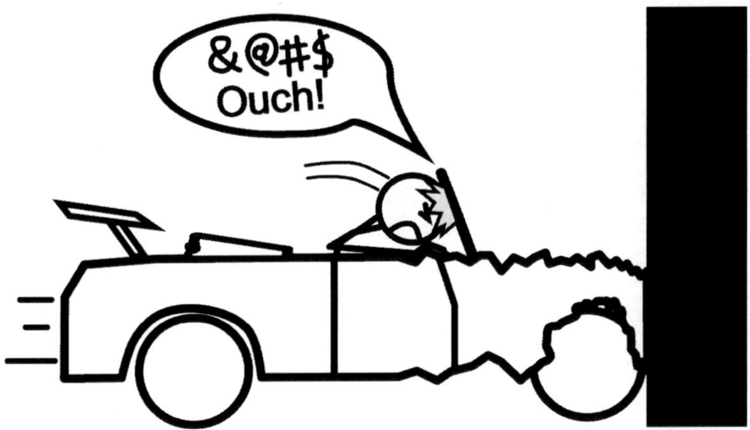

Back to injuries that you can repair. When you're working out to get fitter or stronger, you will often hear the saying: *No pain, no gain.* This is very true! However, in my opinion a more beneficial version of this mantra is

No pain, no gain,
but don't overtrain.

If you are hurting your muscles faster than they can heal and doing it repetitively, you are causing an injury that may never fully heal. Pushing through the pain is what gets you in trouble. If you're feeling some doubt as you read this (*But surely*, you think, *Not pushing through the pain is a sign of weakness!*), you are not alone. This is what we are usually taught in childhood. So, let's find out why pushing through the pain can be a spectacularly bad idea.

Full Repair & Upgrade

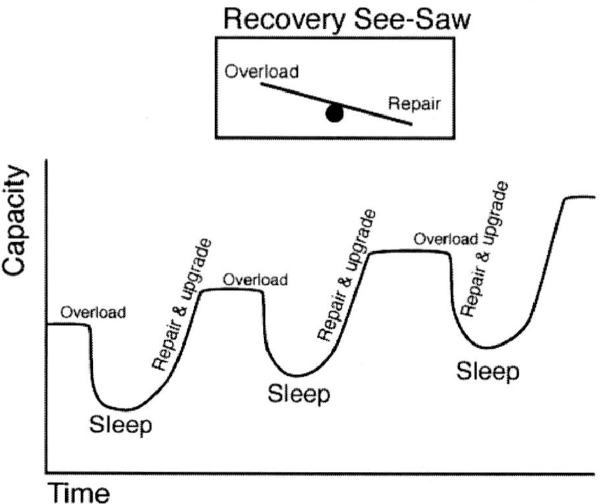

Incomplete Repair - Overtraining

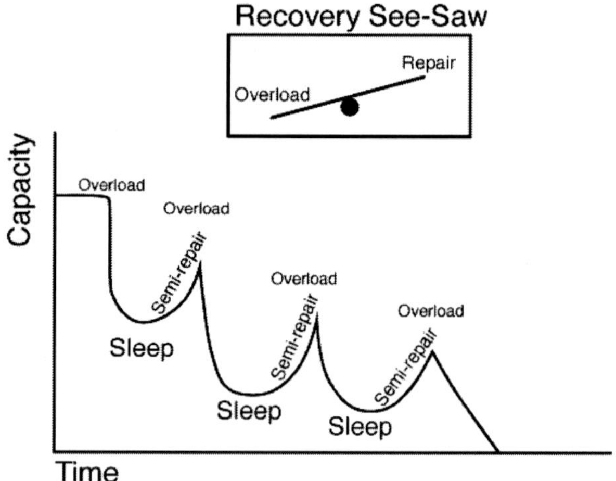

Hitting Your Thumb with a Hammer

I like using the example of hitting your thumb with a hammer to demonstrate what happens when you cause an overload injury. Imagine you're trying to hammer a nail into a piece of wood, and you whack your thumb by accident.

You can tell overload has happened to your thumb because it hurts straight away. The size of the injury can be determined by how much it hurts. Generally, the greater the pain, the greater the injury. The greater the injury, the longer the repair program needs to run for. A gentle tap may feel better in seconds or minutes. A harder hit causes a bruise and will take a couple of days to repair. If you really smash your thumb, hard enough to break a bone, the repair program will take around six weeks. Finally, if the injury is big enough, if you crush your thumb with a sledgehammer, it may not return to the way it was before. After all, there are a lot of carpenters out there with funny-shaped thumbs.

Let's say that in this example, you whack your thumb, and the pain doesn't go away immediately. It sticks around to remind you that your thumb is injured and under repair. Despite the persistent throb, you decide to keep working because you want to get your project done. *Wham!* You hit your thumb again, and more pain pulses through it. Even though it wasn't as hard a hit as the first time, it feels agonizing. You decide to call it a day.

Why did it hurt more the second time you hit your thumb? Because, if you repeat the overload before the repair has finished, the injures add together. This means that

Repetitive overload leads to increasing injury.

If you hit your thumb again, and again, and again, your thumb becomes increasing painful and sensitive. Long-term problems can arise from repeated injury.

In the orthopedic clinic, we deal with countless examples of overload every day. When I treat a patient with a broken leg, I test whether it has healed by pushing on the broken bone and asking if it hurts. I primarily want to make sure they are healed and can therefore use their injured area without pain. If they still feel pain, I recommend being in the cast for another couple of weeks until the pain has improved or gone away. I know that using a painful leg may result in the bone taking longer to heal or even worse, not healing at all.

You can think of healing after you train as "recovery" and overtraining as "incomplete recovery." Another way I talk about this is choosing between Plan A and Plan B. Plan A is repair-and-upgrade mode, and it's where you want to stay. Keep pushing through pain, and you risk going from Plan A to Plan B, which is rescue-repair mode. Just as an athlete can overtrain by trying to improve too much, too soon, you can overtrain any part of your body by trying to change things too quickly. In Part 3, we will consider some of the ways that overtraining and forcing a shift into Plan B can cause a lot of trouble, and what to do when that happens.

PART 3

Understanding Pain

Chapter 15

TOO MUCH OVERLOAD

It is likely that you picked up this book to learn more about ongoing discomfort and pain in your body. Now that you understand the main principles of your body, the nature of overload and efficiency, and why your body responds the way it does to overload, you can apply these concepts to your personal experience with injury and healing.

In this part of the book, we will explore incomplete or failed repair, ongoing issues like chronic pain, gaining unwanted weight, deconditioning, the role that medications play in treating injury and pain, and finally, the consequences of repetitive overload over months and years.

The Four Levels of Overload

To begin, remember that each system has a finite capacity to do work before overload and damage occurs. This means that if you stay within the capacity of the system, no damage is done. If you stretch a system beyond its capacity, some level of overload happens. But how much? Any system can be overloaded, but we'll stick with my favourite example from the musculoskeletal system: hitting your thumb with a hammer.

You want to build a wooden doghouse for your dog, and you call your buddy over to help you. Together you make a plan, buy the wood, gather your tools, and begin. All is going well until you whack your thumb with a hammer. From Part 2, we know that the harder you hit your thumb, the more it hurts and the bigger the injury. The bigger the injury, the longer the inflammation healing program must run to fix it. Remember that your pain stays switched on to protect your thumb while it's under repair. I'm going to use this example to illustrate the four levels of overload you might experience.

Scenario 1: Minor Capacity Overload

You hit your thumb and yelp. Your friend laughs at you. When you experience a minor overload, you feel immediate aching in the affected area that improves in minutes to hours. Minor overload is very common. If your body were a car, this would be the equivalent of getting a scratch in your paint or a flat tire – something that can be repaired quickly and completely.

You give your thumb a good rub and notice that it is a bit redder than usual. It's not a cause for concern, so you continue working on the doghouse with minor pain that eventually fades away.

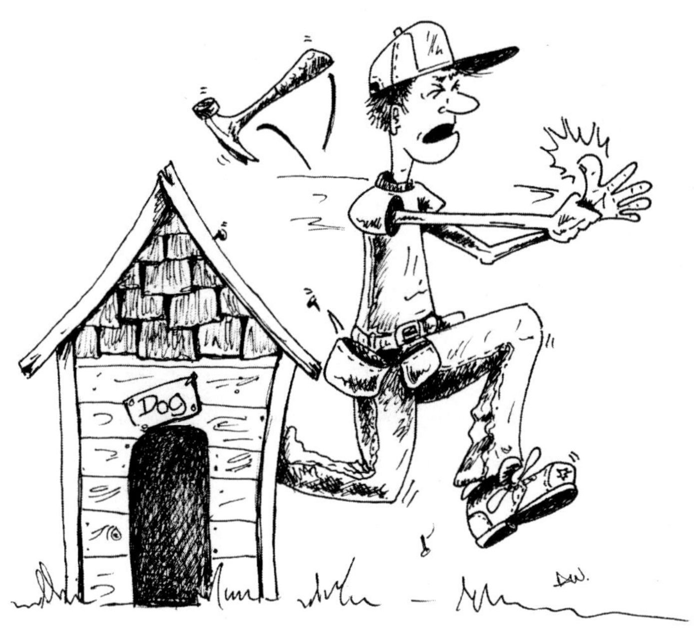

Scenario 2: Moderate Capacity Overload

You hit your thumb, drop the hammer, and shriek, "****ing ouch! You $#@*ing hammer!" Your buddy laughs at you. He posts the video on YouTube and gets a thousand views.

This time, your thumb is quite sore and you can already tell it's going to swell up. When you experience a moderate overload, you feel immediate aching, this time for longer than a few hours. You may continue to work today, but it will be uncomfortable and awkward as you try not to use your thumb. Within an hour or two, your thumb is swollen and sporting a fine plum-coloured bruise.

If your body were a car, this would be the equivalent of wearing out your brakes, getting a minor ding in the bodywork, or cracking your windshield. The damage is more significant but can be completely repaired. Your pain in this case may last a day or two while it heals.

Scenario 3: Major Capacity Overload

"My &*@%ing thumb! Call a ****ing ambulance! What sort of a @#$% friend are you, anyway! Why did you let me %$#*ing do that? Son of a @#$%. Put down your ****ing phone and help me!" Your buddy instead posts a video, and it goes viral.

When you experience a major overload, you feel immediate pain that persists for more than a few days. Hit your thumb hard enough to break the bone, and you'll feel a lot of pain. Once your friend stops laughing, he sees that something more serious has happened, makes a homemade splint for your thumb, and drives you to the hospital.

The repair time for a major overload can range from a couple of days to six weeks, a time during which your pain will persist to discourage you from using your thumb. Your doctor will create a better splint, which prevents movement and facilitates a completed repair.

If your body were a car, this would be the equivalent of engine damage, or a major collision requiring a rebuild. This is when prolonged incomplete repair is a risk; essentially, without proper treatment and repair, this could become an injury that never fully repairs back to its original state, instead receiving a "patch repair" that I'll describe shortly.

Scenario 4: Catastrophic Capacity Overload

"………….. oh." Your buddy puts down his phone. Nobody wants to see this.

When you experience catastrophic overload, you know right away that something bad has happened, and so does your buddy. He doesn't laugh – in fact, he immediately looks away, feeling light-headed. If you completely squash your thumb, it's likely that your injury cannot fully heal. This means that your thumb may always be a funny shape. If you destroy your thumb, a surgeon may decide to amputate it rather than try to repair it.

Catastrophic overload means a significant loss of function in the injured area and ongoing pain that persists until the repair cycle has finished. Importantly, completed repair at this stage may not be possible without external help and may lead to permanent, irreparable damage. For example, some ligaments and muscles may need to be surgically reattached to bones. Broken bones may need to be set straight with a cast or surgically held in a good position with metal. The repair, if it happens, will probably take between two and twelve weeks or more, and the system is unlikely to ever return to its original condition.

If your body were a car, catastrophic overload means that it has been in a major collision. Anyone whose vehicle has been in a major car accident will know that once their car is repaired, it may still function and be generally safe, but there is always something a bit different or not quite right about it. Parts of the car often fail before you expect them to.

In the worst cases, catastrophic overload in the body can lead to a complete loss of function. Scar tissue predominates to hold the system together but in a non-functioning state. With the help of this patch repair your body will adapt to work around the injury, but the system is permanently damaged, as is often seen in spinal cord injuries. This is where comparisons to a car end, because while you can purchase a brand-new car, you cannot get a brand-new body.

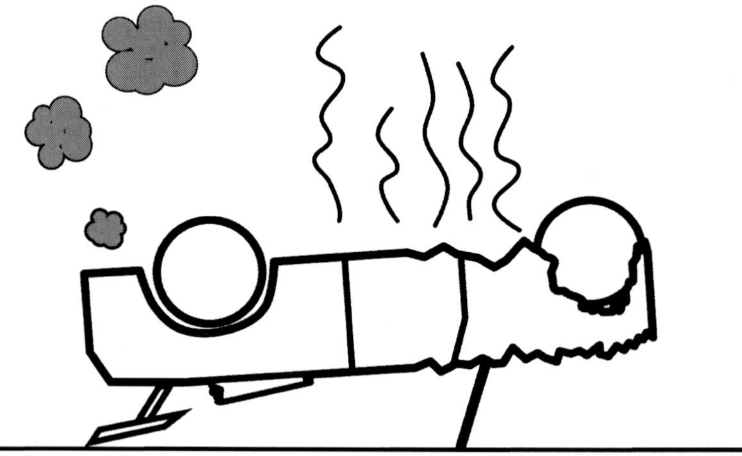

Plan A and Plan B

It is possible after any injury to push through the pain and cause more damage, if you choose to ignore what the pain is telling you. This means running on a sore knee, exposing a residual sunburn to the sun, or hitting your injured thumb with a hammer again. Let's revisit the hammer story to find out what happens when you push through the pain.

If you hit your thumb with a hammer, your body will try to fix what you have done, regardless of the level of overload. Repair mostly happens when you sleep at night. If you wake up and your body hasn't yet fixed the injury, you will still have pain.

Let's say two days after the incident, your thumb is still hurting. However, the doghouse remains unfinished. You wake up early and notice storm clouds on the horizon. *I'd better get this done*, you think, rubbing your thumb. You gather your tools and start hammering away, trying desperately to get the roof finished when – *WHAM* – you hit your thumb again. "#@$%&*!!," you scream.

In Part 2, you learned what happens to your pain when you hit your thumb a second time; it hurts even more, because you have added a new injury to the residual injury that hadn't finished its repair cycle. You don't have to hit it hard; you just have to hit it again.

Something else happens when you do this. Your body begins to suspect that this repair might be more expensive than it planned for, as the same injury keeps happening before it finishes repairing. Your body has a decision to make now: try to quickly complete the repair and upgrade the area again *or* treat this injury as a failed repair: Plan A or Plan B.

Once you have caused overload in your system more than once, it's easy to get trapped in a "failed repair cycle" because *it takes very little effort to cause more damage*. You can stop repair or cause more damage simply by doing what you've always done, or even by doing less than usual but still too much in the context of your injury. At this time pushing through the pain is the worst thing to do. In other words:

All you need to do to maintain an injury is hurt yourself more than you are healing yourself.

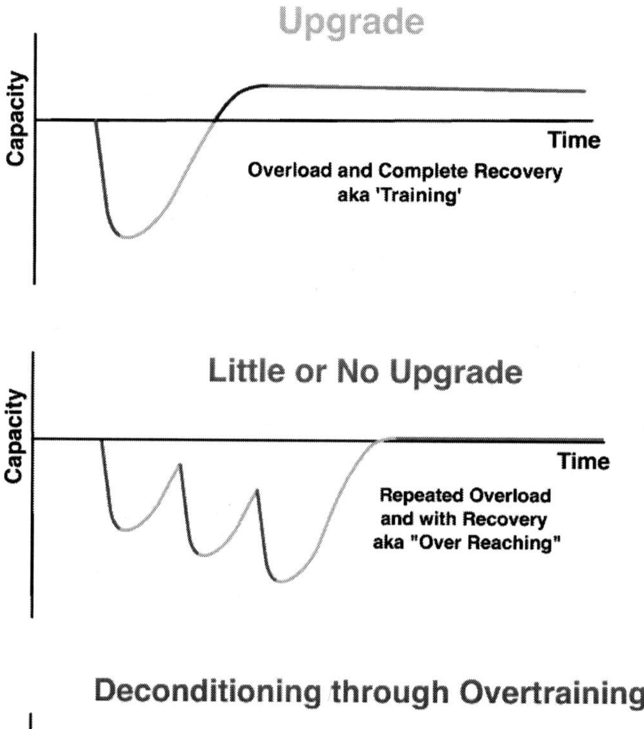

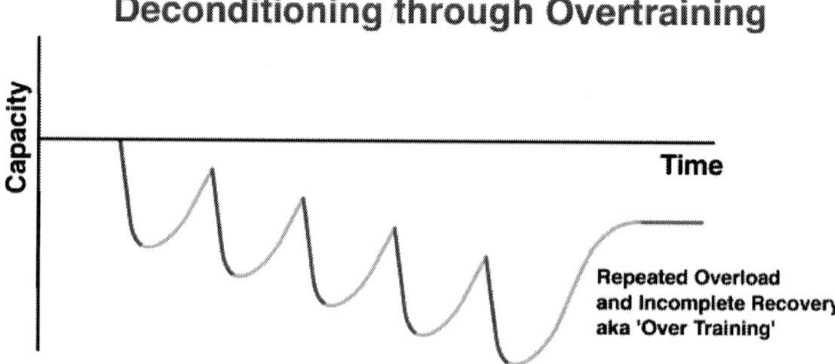

Remember, when a system is damaged and needs to be repaired, its capacity to do its job is greatly reduced. This makes repeated overload injuries much more likely. For example, tearing a knee ligament, such as your anterior cruciate ligament (ACL), is a common catastrophic overload. Your knee swells up and aches, you experience pain, limited range of motion, and weakness, and it hurts a lot to put weight on it.

What's So Bad about Pushing through the Pain?

You take a week or two off to recover but want to get back to activity, as you are normally an active person. Before you hurt your knee, you regularly walked 3 km a day. You feel you've given your knee long enough to heal so you head out on your regular walk and decide to push through the pain. After 500 m your knee starts to hurt but you think, *no pain, no gain,* and push on. At 1 km you pop a couple of pain pills and decide to call it a day.

You may be able to take painkillers and still go for a 1 km walk; however, given the newly decreased capacity of your knee, even this reduced distance will significantly overload it. This overload will lead to further injury, which means that the next day when you push it and go for another walk, you might only make it 500 m, which is enough to cause another overload injury. After a few days of pushing it, walking from room to room becomes difficult. Ultimately, repetitive overload can lead to a failure of your body to complete its healing cycle at all.

The inflammation program has an important role here. When you hurt yourself, your body tries to fix your overloaded system as fast as it can. This fast-repair mode is called "acute inflammation." The acute inflammation program is very expensive for your body because it uses a lot of resources, but it also fixes your system *quickly* and tries to give you an upgrade to prevent you from hurting yourself again. This is Plan A.

Your body has a second repair mode, Plan B, which is reserved for situations when Plan A is not allowed to finish – in other words, when you injure yourself again (hit your thumb more times or walk on your injured knee) before your system has time to repair. Plan B is not ideal. When there is an imbalance between healing and repair that goes on for long enough, it becomes too expensive to try to repair your system quickly. Plan B can also be called "chronic inflammation" and is a clever way for your body to fix things as *cheaply* as possible when fixing things as *quickly* as possible is no longer an option. The problem with Plan B is that it takes a very long time and does not lead to an upgrade. Plan A generally takes six to twelve weeks. Plan B can take months to years.

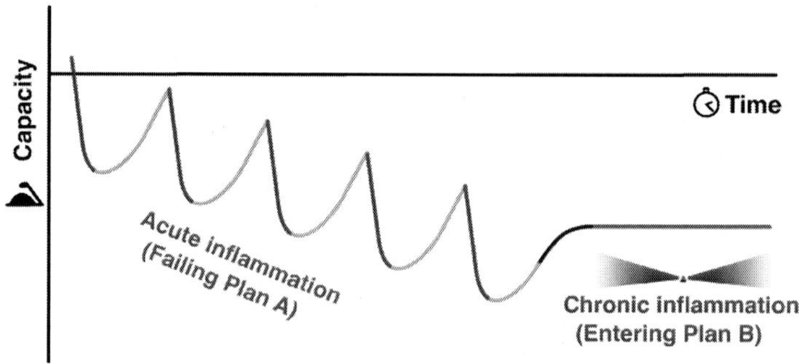

Repetitively overloading without time to fully repair

The War of Overload

When describing overload, acute inflammation, and chronic inflammation, I like to use the example of fighting a war. Inflammation, after all, is your body's universal emergency service that arrives to fix problems.

At the first sign of war, a country (in this case, your body) musters the biggest army and all the resources it can and orders them to the battlefield in a full-frontal assault in hopes of winning the conflict quickly. This is the equivalent of Plan A. It's a very expensive strategy, but it can have great results. After all, if you respond faster with better resources and more infantry than the enemy, you'll overpower them and win. In terms of an injury, Plan A can result in completed repair and victory.

However, if you lose that first battle, you must try again. Attempt number two (think of every war movie you've ever watched) involves gathering your remaining infantry and resources, delivering a deeply moving speech, and ordering another charge. This is your inflammation rushing back into the battlefield, throwing everything it has at the problem to try to fix it quickly.

If you charge a few more times and *fail*, you'll probably look around at the remains of your army and decide that it's a bad strategy to take another run at the enemy. You need to save your remaining resources and keep the enemy at bay in a new way. In an inflammatory sense, this means that your body recognizes that with these repetitive overloads and failed attempts at repair, completed repair is unlikely to happen.

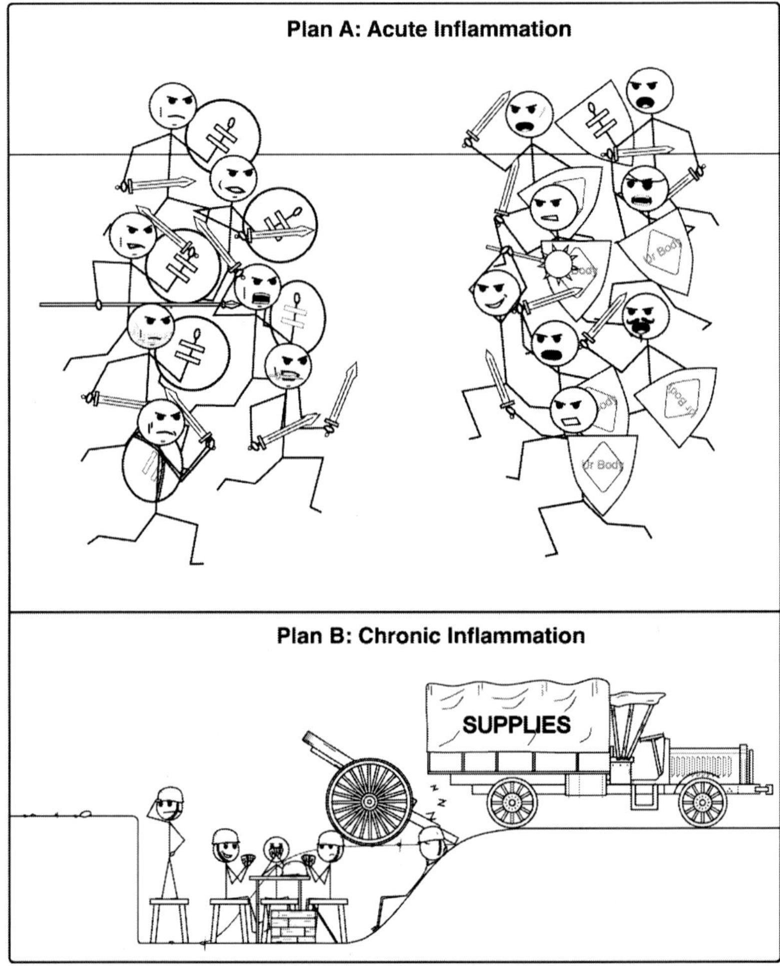

It's time to change tactics to Plan B. In a war, this usually means digging in. You stop trying full frontal assaults and start digging trenches and building walls. The tactic changes to *a war of attrition*. You set up a supply chain of resources and infrastructure that will help you win the battle slowly or at least keep the enemy at bay. With this strategy the enemy will have more difficulty crossing your line of defense and you can decrease the number of infantries required to maintain your border. After all, you need your precious resources for other things, like keeping your home industries running.

In your body, this means that acute inflammation (Plan A) is abandoned *even though the repair was never completed*. Plan B starts when your body decides to fix things slowly and more cheaply so that it can prioritize other important body functions. Pain and repair go together. If the repair cannot be completed in Plan A and your body enters plan B, your pain goes on for longer than expected (longer than twelve weeks and maybe even for years). In a war sense, you failed to win quickly and are now under siege. The enemy is outside your gates and requires your ongoing attention. *You learn to live in war time*. This is rarely a good experience.

When you enter chronic inflammation (Plan B), a few things happen. Just like hitting your thumb repeatedly with a hammer, you feel pain in that area more easily. Increased sensitivity is your body's attempt to prevent you from causing more injury. As your pain lingers and increases, you will likely move less or differently to avoid the pain. While this protects your injured system to some extent, you start to decondition the parts of your body that you aren't using. As you decondition, the possibility of overload increases as your capacity decreases. It's a vicious cycle.

Usually, after months up to a couple of years of siege, the war suddenly ends. Most people leave the wasteland behind as the conflict is over. However, for some people, even though the war is done and things are quiet again, they are so used to war-time living that they can't stop living this way. In your body, this means Plan B is over, but the pain goes on without more input. This sensitization is called "chronic pain." Your body keeps reporting on a problem even though it is over. I call this Plan B+. More on this later, in Chapter 18.

How to Avoid the Cycle of Failed Repair

If you have experienced an overload injury, but have not entered the vicious cycle of failed repair, there are a few important things you can do to heal completely:

1. Let your body complete its repair (Plan A) and allow acute inflammation to finish its job. Depending on the injury, this could be one night, three months, or sometimes more.

2. Seek external help if the injury requires it (e.g., go to the hospital) and follow the protocols for repair, allowing it to heal as fully as it can. Injuries heal predictably but this may be the first time you have experienced this injury. Navigating solo can be a frightening experience. Health care professionals have a wealth of experience with managing injuries just like yours.

3. Take a break. Remember that while it's in repair mode, your system's capacity is greatly reduced. During this important stage, causing repetitive overload is easier than you think. Do not try to strengthen or push the injured area beyond its capacity before it has completed its repair. How can you do this? Listen to your body's feedback: The pain you feel. Pain is your body trying to help you. It is not trying to spoil your fun but rather help you heal fully so you don't hurt yourself more. Returning to work too soon is a very common cause for prolonging or preventing complete healing. When the pain is gone, your repair cycle has completed.

4. Maximize healing capacity. Avoid causing overload in other systems while the injured system is in repair mode. Your body is always prioritizing what needs attention and will allocate resources to high-priority systems. This means that an injury in a low-priority system will get fewer resources or won't complete the repair at all if a high-priority system is under attack. Smoking is a great example of this, one that we will talk more about. Damaging your guts with alcohol or junk food won't help either.

5. Give your body what it needs to repair. Eat healthy, nutritious food and get a lot of sleep while you are healing. We will talk more about optimizing healing in Part 5!

6. Take time to recondition. When you have a reduced level of functioning, your body will efficiently decondition anything that is not being used while healing. As you recover, return to previous activities slowly. You must listen to your body, not your boss or the coach! To quote one of the surgeons I work with:

"Start low, slow and easy."

or my version is:

Low and slow is the way to go.

The original injury is repaired but now you must slowly retrain your deconditioned body. More on this in Part 5 as well.

But what happens if you are already caught in the cycle of failed repair? If you still feel pain for something that should have healed long ago and now you realize that you have been repeatedly overloading your system for a while, what can you do?

Chapter 16

YOUR BODY'S "PLAN B"

Chronic inflammation opens you up to a cycle of increasing and persistent pain, limited capacity, and body adaptations because of the pain. If you're nodding along, I don't need to tell you how frustrating and exhausting this is. Chronic inflammation happens most commonly in leg and back injuries because it's very hard to stop walking or using your back even with simple activities. Pain sticks around to remind you not to overload the damaged system. However, even after weeks, months, or years, the pain *should* eventually resolve if the repair process can complete to the best of its ability. The problem is that sometimes it doesn't. We will talk about the move from chronic inflammation to chronic pain later but first let's talk a bit more about Plan B.

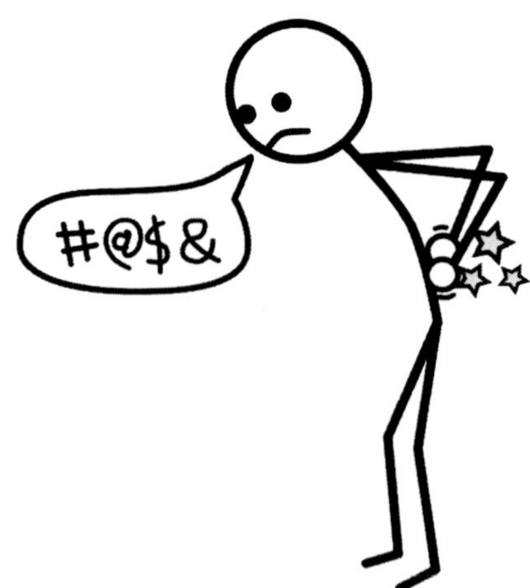

Minor Injuries with Catastrophic Consequences

Failed repair is not unique to major and catastrophic injuries. In fact, the commonest failed repair injuries are minor "repetitive strain injuries" (RSI), which occur when you cause a minor overload over and over again. Sometimes trivial overload injuries can have devastating consequences. Say you go for a hike with some friends. During the hike you twist your ankle, and your only choice is to walk back to the parking lot. Each time you overload your injured ankle by stepping on it, you increase the injury. This results in an escalating injury with a repair cycle that will take longer to complete.

If you injure your ankle a few metres from the parking lot, your journey to the car takes a couple of minutes and your overload injury is only minor. The required repair cycle will be short. If you're a couple of kilometres away from the parking lot, you'll likely get back to your car with no more than a moderate overload and drive home, recovering in a couple of days. However, if you need to walk 10 km back to your car, you will arrive back at your car a few hours later, limping, your minor injury now a moderate or even major one. The required repair cycle will be much longer.

Imagine how much this situation escalates when you twist your ankle alone, 20 km from your car! It is now very likely to become a significant injury before you get back. It might even cost you your life if you can't walk anymore. In other words, a sprained ankle would not normally kill you, but given the right circumstances, it could.

Another common example of minor repetitive overload leading to chronic inflammation is overtraining for a sport.

This is when the no-pain,-no-gain mentality sets in. Say you're training to run a half marathon. You start off bold and manage to run 8 km on the first day. By the time you get home, your knees ache. You spend a day limping around. The next day, when they feel a little better, you decide to run the same distance again despite lingering pain. This is called "over-reaching" (training again before you have fully recovered). You consider pushing yourself to be a sign of mental strength and determination. You pat yourself on the back.

Your knees are still complaining a few days after the second run, so you take pain medication and keep to your plan, belligerently increasing your run to 12 km. You carry on this way for a few weeks leading up to your race. At this point, it doesn't matter whether you finish the race or not; the important thing is that during this time, the repair cycle *never completed* from that first injury. You have now overtrained. For weeks, you simply allowed your overload injury to repair *just enough* for you to ignore the pain and overload it again. Once the race is over, you feel heightened pain and decide to take a break from running. But even though you stop running completely, the pain does not go away.

In the workplace, two common examples of repetitive strain injuries are overusing a computer mouse and sitting in a chair that forces you into poor posture. Using a computer mouse might seem like a trivial activity until you repeat it thousands of times in a day. This small activity can add up to a lot of work for your arm and start to make it ache. If you are overloading during the day more than you are repairing at night, you will be slowly accumulating a bigger injury over time. Sitting too long in a chair can have a similar effect on your back. In fact, this is how many persistent aches and pains "develop" over months and years.

These are not dramatic injuries. However, the resulting accumulated overload can be huge. A seemingly innocent activity has resulted in an injury causing significant, persistent pain. You have pushed your body into Plan B. Your pain may feel like it's never improving, even months after your hike, your race, or buying a new chair. The consequences can be catastrophic if you lose your job or have to stop doing what you love.

Why People with the Same Problem Experience Different Pain

For years, something puzzled me in my practice. I was working with many patients who presented similar amounts of wear and tear but different outcomes. I asked myself, and my colleagues, questions like: *Why do two people have an equally bad-looking knee X-ray, but one has dreadful pain and the other doesn't?* My colleagues didn't have a clear answer either. How could two people's knees be equally worn out, but their pain experiences be so different? When I applied the concept of repetitive overload and unfinished repair attempts, the answer became clearer.

Say two people have the same degree of wear and tear in their knees. We call this osteoarthritis, which is pain caused by a joint wearing out. The changes in osteoarthritis that we can see on an X-ray are predictable, but the pain from these changes is difficult to predict and varies from person to person. However, we might have more insight now.

Suppose one person's knee has been *repetitively overloaded without proper repair time* and the pain has never gone away. Meanwhile, a second person with a similar injury *allowed their repair cycle to finish*. This means that even with an identical X-ray to the first person, the second person feels less pain, and the pain goes away. The capacity of their knee has even increased, as they have learned to stay within the capacity of their knee and its ability to repair.

Allowing your repair cycle to complete makes all the difference.

It doesn't matter how worn out or broken things are. Your body always has a plan to try to make things better.

Because of this, it's quite common to meet patients with the same degree of knee osteoarthritis where one person can barely walk up the stairs and the other goes skiing every weekend.

Why Is Pain Hard to Predict?

Pain is confusing. You've probably heard of someone who injured themselves terribly but reported no pain, and another who experienced a lot of pain from a small injury. Perhaps you've experienced this yourself; it's frustrating to meet someone with a similar problem who experiences much less pain and fewer consequences than you.

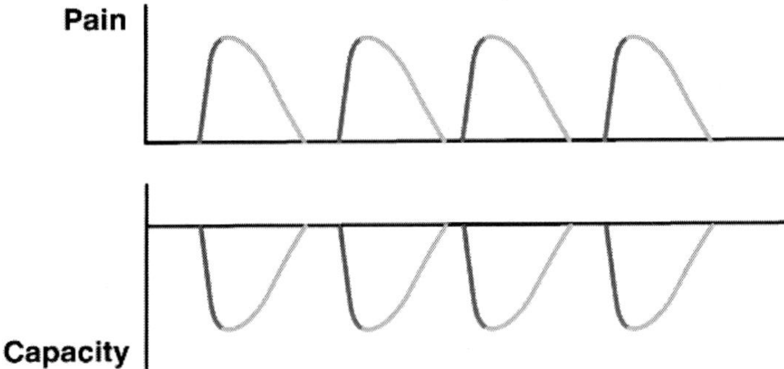

Functional load and full recovery
"Manageable pain with osteoarthritis"

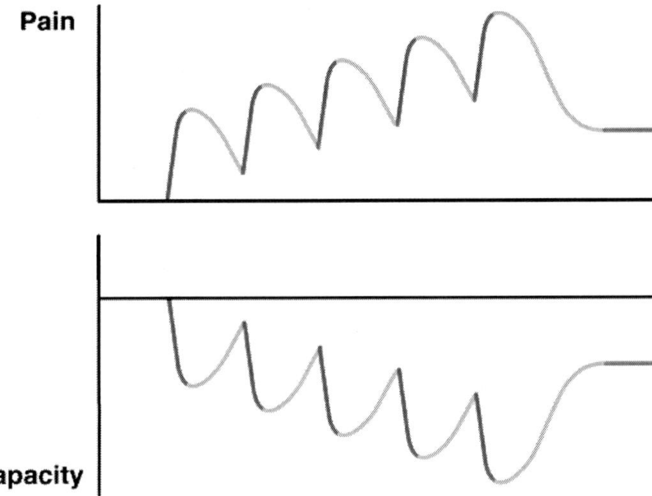

Overtraining in osteoarthritis
"Escalating pain and decreasing functional capacity"

The tear and repair (or failed repair) cycle goes some way to explaining why people experience different levels of pain for the same injury. However, it's not the full story. How you experience pain is complicated because the way your body reports pain can be turned up or down. Your pain is modulated by many factors, and the pain signal can be changed, depending on what else is going on in your body. Some factors modulating the pain response include

1. Other injuries your body is repairing: Your body tells you about the most important thing going on at any moment in time. If you have two problems, it only tells you about the worst one. This is called "gating." We will talk more about gating in the next chapter.

2. Your emotional state: This is a big topic, and one which we will explore later in more depth. It's important to note that the relationship between emotions, memories, and pain is one that we still know very little about! However, there is general agreement that emotions greatly impact why, how, and when we feel pain.

3. Nerve modulation: Nerves can be sensitized or desensitized. The most common example of nerves being sensitized is when they "learn" to get better at reporting a regularly occurring pain signal. Once you learn to feel pain, your body tends to over report it. More on this in the next chapters.

The nerve itself may also be damaged. Just like a faulty wire in your car's electrics, this can lead to "faulty signals." If you squeeze or damage a nerve, it reports this with a pain signal. For example, with sciatica, you may get pain that goes from your back all the way down your leg to your foot. It can feel like a foot problem, but the actual problem is the trapping and squeezing of the nerve in your back that goes to your foot. This pain then "radiates" down to your foot and it may feel like your foot is injured. The pain signal for "squeezed sciatic nerve in your back" and "damaged foot" can feel the same. At first, this irritated nerve may become sensitized and simply over report already existing problems in your foot. If the nerve is damaged more, the pain may worsen. With continued damage, the nerve may become "desensitized" as it stops working completely. This results in numbness and even weakness, as the nerve stops doing its job.

The faulty reporting of pain signals can make interpreting pain even more confusing. Imagine have an intermittent wiring problem in your car or your house. These wiring issues can be challenging to figure out.

Navigating Pain Is a Challenge

You have learned about Plan A (quick but expensive repair) and Plan B (slow and cheap repair that doesn't lead to an upgrade). You know that if Plan A does not complete the repair, your body goes into Plan B. With that said:

The pain signal you experience in Plan A and Plan B <u>can feel the same</u>.

This makes pain very confusing. It is difficult to know if you are in Plan A or Plan B by simply experiencing pain. To provide a real-life example, let's return to hitting your thumb with a hammer. When you hit your thumb, it hurts! It continues to hurt until your body finishes healing. This is a straightforward mechanism unless you repetitively injure your thumb and go into Plan B, which causes the pain to linger for longer. There is no obvious signal telling you that you have crossed the threshold from acute pain (Plan A) to chronic inflammation (Plan B). All you know is that your thumb still hurts.

Once you have pain that does not go away after about three months, the pain signals seem less useful, and you have most likely entered plan B. The injured part of your body either hurts all the time or hurts easily when you use it. In this state, when you ask yourself what your pain is trying to tell you, you may conclude that your body just hates you or that something bad has happened.

If your pain persists for years, you feel like your body really hates you. This is when you have entered Plan B+ or chronic pain. The pain has gone on longer than everyone expected and now people are telling you that you "shouldn't have this pain" anymore. How we define these pain states is based mostly on expected timings of healing.

Healing Mode	Plan	Injury	Pain	Length	Resolution	Examples
Acute Inflammation	Plan A	Under repair	Resolves with healing	Days to months	Completed repair	Any injury
Chronic Inflammation	Plan B	Failed repair	Persists but eventually goes away	Months to years	Failed repair program completed	RSI, over-training, frozen shoulder, plantar fasciitis, tennis elbow, ongoing back pain
Chronic Pain	Plan B+	Pain sensi-tisation	Persistent pain, no end point	Years	None	Whiplash, chronic regional pain syndrome,nerve damage

Table 1 – Healing modes

Interpreting your pain is an important role of doctors.

A doctor's job is to determine whether the pain you are experiencing is signalling that you need external help. Doctors are trained to recognize what's going on by examining and testing what your body is doing. They have learned to recognize the stories your body is telling them to make a diagnosis.

It can be difficult for someone suffering from pain to understand what their body is telling them on their own. For example, not all chest pain signals a heart attack. Two people having chest pain will respond differently based on other injuries they are dealing with at the same time, their emotional state (which can be informed by their past experiences with chest pain), and their unique nerve modulation. Importantly, some chest pain *does* indicate a heart attack, which is why doctors don't mess around with chest pain. If you report it, they urgently investigate your pain and respond accordingly.

As pain can be confusing, learning about how and why your body reports pain to you is a key part of understanding your body's language. We will now think more about how your body tells you about what it is up to. Not all information is important all of the time. Let's look at how your body presents its latest "up to the minute" situational report.

Chapter 17

SENSATION AND EMOTION GATING

What do you really need to know in order to run your body? From moment to moment, you are not aware of every heartbeat, muscle twitch, digestive process, or even every pain. This is for a very good reason.

Imagine you are transported into the cockpit of a space rocket and find yourself lying back in the astronaut's pilot seat. The capsule is lit by a dizzying array of hundreds of blinking lights, and you are surrounded by dozens of switches and gauges. It is up to you to pilot this thing! How do you know which one of these lights and gauges needs your attention right now?

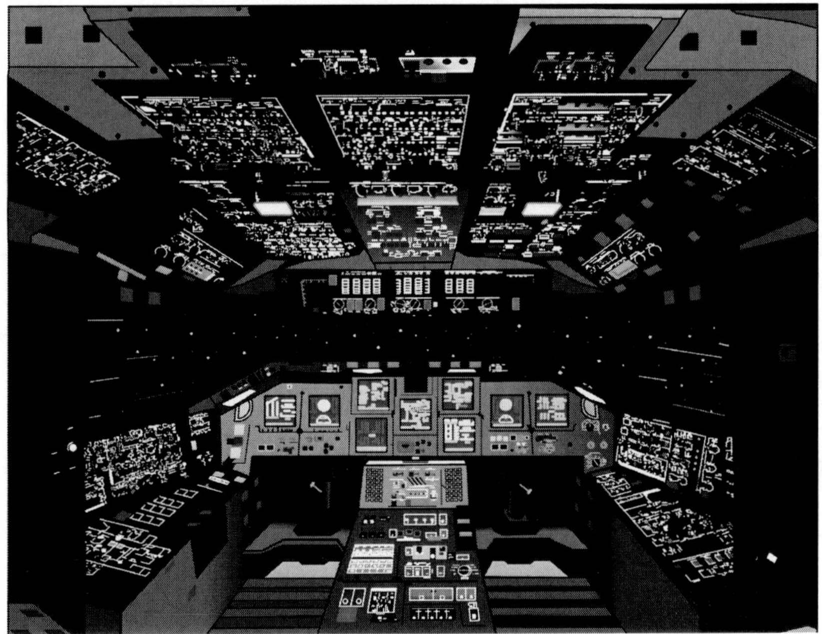

Your body is just as complex as this space rocket, with just as many signals. To help you determine what to pay attention to, your body does a neat trick. It simply turns on the most important "light," or sensation, at any moment in time. It may cycle through lights quickly as each light's information becomes more important than the last. All you have to do is act on the most important light. Once you have dealt with what it is telling you and it switches off, the next most important thing lights up.

This filtering of information is called gating. According to gating theory, any sensation in your body must get through a gate to come to your attention. A lot of the available information is not allowed through and is "gated out." This means that although your body may experience hundreds of sensations at a time, only one sensation is reported at a time. This process probably happens in your spinal cord and brain.

Imagine two sensations arrive at your spinal cord at the same time. They are like two messengers trying to squeeze through a wooden gate. Only one of the messengers is allowed through the gate at a time, so even though your body registers both sensations it only tells you the most important one. This means that although you may feel pain in your hand, foot, and head after a fall, this is because you can cycle between these sensations extremely quickly. You are truly only aware of one sensation at a time.

Test it! The next time you have a pain (like a headache), try creating a bigger pain by pinching the webbing between your thumb and index finger. Squeeze hard until this pain is greater than your other pain and see what happens to the first pain. Stop squeezing and your first pain will come back.

Why Does Your Body Gate Out Information?

You may already have guessed the answer to this question. That's right, it's our old friend, efficiency! It is not efficient for you to deal with all the available information at once. To ensure you do the most important thing, your body brings attention to the most pressing matter at hand.

Let's say you stumble across a bear in the woods. Your body will help you escape this dangerous situation by suppressing or gating information that isn't going to help you. While running away, you will not feel hungry even if you're starving, and you will be able to run even if your ankle is hurting. Your body is trying to save itself from very expensive damage or even death. To do this it only sends the feedback that you need in order to escape.

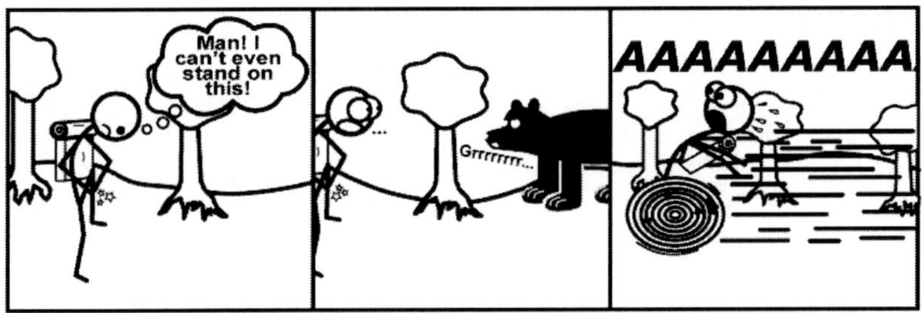

Your body's fight-or-flight response can override everything to make sure you can get out of there ASAP!

Here are some other examples of your body prioritizing sensations:

- Your hearing becomes more sensitive in the dark to compensate for impaired vision
- Your sense of taste and smell increase when you are hungry
- If you injure yourself during intense sport, you may not feel it until afterwards

We can also look at this another way, which is noticing what we *don't feel* normally. For example:

- You are not aware of your heart beating until it starts to beat too fast, and you get "palpitations"
- You are not aware of your guts working unless they become stretched from eating too much food, and you get a belly ache
- You are not aware of breathing until you hold your breath underwater or run so hard that you are gasping for air
- You are not aware of needing to pee until your bladder is full

Hierarchy of Priorities

When it comes to gating sensations, your body has a hierarchical list in which it ranks the importance of sensations, one over another. This allows it to send you the most important information when a lot of things are going on at once. Interestingly, pain is not at the top of this list. The priority list for your body's sensations appears to go as follows:

1. Touch sensation allows you to feel sensations as subtle as a soft breeze. It also makes you sensitive to dangerous things, like feeling the side of your heel slip over the edge of a cliff, or the sensation of a red ant crawling on your arm. Touch sensation gives you the most important information about the world and helps you navigate it.

2. Temperature sensation allows you to discern between heat and cold. We are warm-blooded, which means our machines operate within a narrow temperature range. Too cold or too hot and our machinery stops working properly or is completely broken. Without a high level of temperature sensation and regulation, you would be more likely to put yourself in life-threatening situations without being aware of the danger.

3. Pain helps you understand when you have overloaded a system and are in a state of repair. This is what we have spent a lot of time on in this book. Notice that pain is not as high on the priority list as touch and temperature. Think about it this way: If you were constantly aware of pain over touch or temperature, you would live a life filled with pain. Since pain is lower on the hierarchy, it means that your body only sends you pain sensations when it is important that you feel them so you can repair.

4. Proprioception is your awareness of how your body is positioned and where it is in space. Proprioception helps you balance and move with ease. It is last in the hierarchy of sensations because it is more important to receive information about an injury than it is to have good balance or positioning. For example, when you sprain your ankle it can feel wobbly, or if you have chronic hip pain your balance can get worse, both happen because your pain is overriding your proprioception. After a joint injury or surgery, it can take a long time until you "trust" your joint again, as it does not feel right.

Can You Use Sensation Gating to Your Advantage?

The short answer is yes! To understand this, let's return to the twisted ankle example. Because touch sensation is prioritized over other sensations, including pain, it means that if you twist your ankle and feel pain, rubbing it makes it feel better. Strapping your ankle also makes it feel better, because the bandage touching the skin creates reassuring pressure that lessens pain.

Temperature sensation is prioritized next, also above pain. If you put a heat or ice pack on your injured ankle, it will also decrease your pain. Touch is still prioritized over temperature, which means that if you rub your ankle after icing it, you will still feel the soothing rubbing sensation even if the skin is a bit numb ... unless you have damaged your nerves by over-icing. Generally, it's a good idea to ice an injury for a maximum of twenty minutes before letting it fully warm up again.

Knowing that proprioception sensation (joint positioning) is prioritized last, below pain, you can understand why your sprained ankle feels wobbly. If you try to stand on it, it hurts and feels unstable as the pain overrides your proprioception. In this case, the pain tells you not to walk on your ankle, because you may overload it again. Feeling wobbly at this stage is nothing to worry about.

When you injure yourself, follow your instincts and use this knowledge to your advantage! After twisting your ankle, take a quiet moment and rub your ankle to lessen your discomfort, bandage it up, and use cold and possibly heat later. The dogma is cold for the first day or two and then heat after that. Importantly, listen to what it's telling you when you start to walk on it again. The pain will tell you how much weight bearing is tolerated.

It's important to note that because of pain gating, you may have more than one injury but not know about it. If the second injury is less severe, it may even go through the whole of the acute pain cycle, or even the chronic pain cycle, without your knowledge. For example, say you have a chronically painful back and you hurt your shoulder while helping a friend move. You may be surprised one day when your doctor looks at a scan of your shoulder and tells you that you have had a problem for years!

Sensations Have Priorities

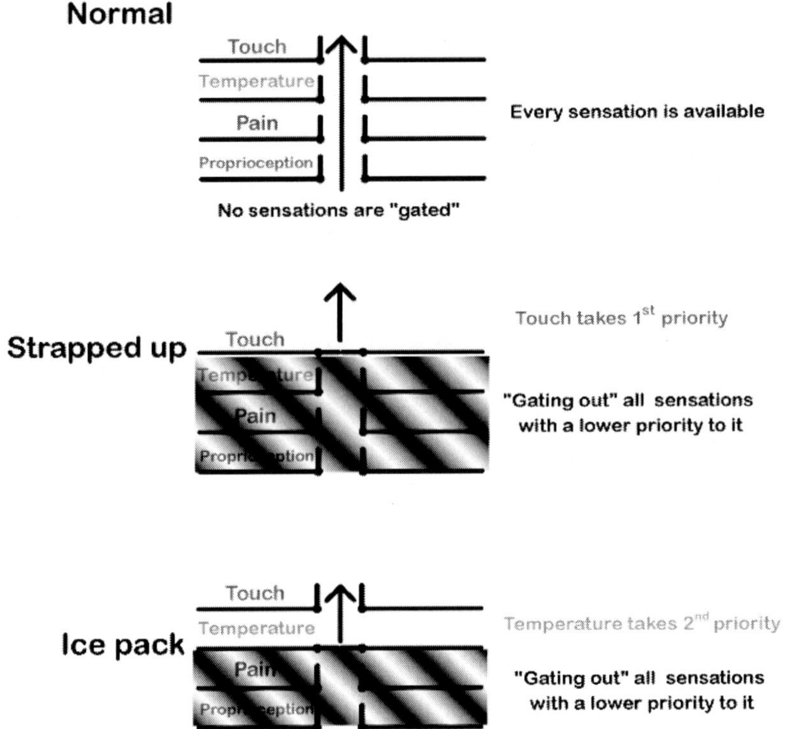

Are Emotions Gated Too?

Emotions impact why, how, and when we feel pain, but this is highly complex and not well understood, even by professionals. When you see that bear in the woods you feel a rush of fear, and that fear is part of why you can forget your hunger and your twisted ankle and run faster than you ever have.

Emotions are your body reporting what your hormones are doing at any one time. Hormones tell your body what mode to be in. For instance, your fight-or-flight response may be triggered by seeing the bear. You suddenly feel extremely motivated to get the **** out of there! This emotional (hormonal) response gates out the other less important emotions that you were feeling before you saw the bear. You are now not aware of how lovely it feels to be in the forest anymore!

Although less predictable than how sensations are prioritized, some emotions seem better at overriding others. For example, being "all loved up" can make you seem irrational as you ignore other emotions. Love seems to be of high priority, with the power to overcome anger.

Hormones can also modulate sensations. For example, adrenalin not only makes you faster and stronger but also sharpens your vision. Seeing that bear makes your senses more active to help you escape. You now see that low-lying branch in the tree and climb to safety. Other sensations can be down-regulated by hormones. The hormones that make you feel in love can decrease pain sensations, which means that pain can be more tolerable when you feel loved and supported.

Anyone who has been in a lot of pain can attest to how emotions impact pain. When I'm in pain I can be a real jerk. Imagine that emotions are paint colours. Love or pleasure is like the colour white. When added to other emotions, it lightens them. Anger is like the colour black. It deepens all the other emotions. Fatigue is like watering down your paint. You feel less of other emotions until you finally fall asleep.

Emotions tell us what our hormones are up to in response to our external circumstances. A long queue at the post office may cause you frustration but speaking with a kind stranger may allow your frustration to be overridden for a bit. In this way, emotions tell you about your body's current state, which again has to do with efficiency.

Your body produces hormones, which cause you to feel emotions that prompt you to respond in a particular way. Your body is encouraging you to behave in a way that is least costly to it in the long run. Anger is a toned-down fight-or-flight response to help you regain control of your circumstances, you feel in love with someone who helps nurture you, you feel hungry when you need food, and so forth.

You are not always aware why this is going on. You just feel a certain way. When you get to the front of the post office queue you may give the clerk behind the desk a hard time, even if you don't know why you feel angry with him. The reason you are angry is that someone cut in on you in the queue. Because this triggered an angry emotion in you, you use this operational state as you interact with the post office clerk. The clerk may wonder: *What have I done to deserve this person being such a jerk?!* You're still operating under the hormonal instructions from your last interaction. Because of this, how you feel is not always a good way to make decisions.

How Does Your Body Prioritize Emotions?

Your body's emotional priorities are unique to you. For example, consider concentrated thought as an emotional state of your body. You may find it easy to get distracted by your thoughts. You may get so lost in thought that you lose all awareness of what is going on around you. How often this happens and how powerfully it happens is unique to you.

If you observe how your body behaves in different circumstances, you can derive a list of emotional priorities unique to you. We will speak more about the role of emotions in the next chapter, but for now, consider that you may habitually respond with some emotions over others, based on your past experiences, beliefs, and values. Here is an example list. Yours will likely be different.

1. Fatigue: This emotion seems to override all others. It dilutes other emotions, and in the end leads to the feeling of needing to shut down and sleep.

2. Fear: This emotion is what shows up when you see a bear. It overrides lesser feelings like hunger or wonder. This is your emergency "get the @$#* out of here" mode. You must be very, very tired to beat this one, but people can still fall asleep in the middle of a war.

3. Pleasure (e.g., love): This emotion allows you to feel forgiving and joyous even in situations that would normally cause you anger or anxiety. Being loved up is a great feeling! Having a laugh is a close second.

4. Analytical thought: This is when you get "lost in thought" and shut out many other emotions and awareness of the world around you. This can be a problem for me. I am frequently asked, "Are you listening to me?"

5. Excitement: This is an emotion that might prompt you to purchase a plane ticket without having planned it, overwhelmed by the promise of freedom and escape. The thrill of the chase!

6. Anger: This emotion can result in ranting at the employee of a big box store for being out of stock of something that was listed as in stock. Often, anger is even pettier than this, but hey, I'm giving you the benefit of the doubt!

7. Anxiety: This emotion is when you feel nervous or uncertain, trying to consider all the possible outcomes. It is closely related to a feeling of losing control of your circumstances.

Can You Use Emotional Prioritizing to Your Advantage?

Just as touch and temperature sensations reduce your pain, you can use your emotions to change your experience. If you have anxiety, you can use pleasure to override it. For example, if you are anxious at the airport, listening to a fun, lighthearted song can ease your anxiety, help you breathe deeper, and remind you that you have plenty of time. Using anger to override anxiety (yelling at the guy who just cut in line in front of you) may also work but replaces a negative emotion with another one.

Overcoming negative emotions by finding a situation or activity you like is called "self-soothing." Self-soothing means inducing a hormonal response that overrides less desirable hormonal responses. For example, you can alter an unpleasant experience by doing something pleasurable instead. Going outside in the sunshine and moving your body can override fear, anger, and anxiety. It is a good idea to have a portfolio of pleasurable activities in your life to help you become aware of, and lift, negative emotional states. I personally find concentrated thought a more powerful analgesic than any pain pill. For example, when I was post-op and having a pain crisis, I wrote a lot of this book! The writing process worked even better than swearing for lessening my anger and pain, although I did a lot of that too!

As your body is reporting the most important piece of information, this can be either a sensation or an emotion. In this way a sensation can gate out an emotion or vice versa. If you are stressed, a massage can help you to relax by focusing you on the sensations of the massage. Going for a run can help clear your head by making you aware of the sensations of being outdoors and using your muscles. Emotions can gate out sensations too. Being engrossed in a movie could stop you feeling your back pain. This interplay between emotions, sensations, and actions will be explored more when we consider changing habits later in the book.

Sleep is also very important to restore your emotions and sensations. While recovering from my surgery, I slept a great deal. If you often find yourself in a state of agitation, impatience, fear, anger, and/or anxiety, take a closer look at your sleep habits. Having a good night's sleep repairs your body and mind. This means that whatever problems or challenges you face today can be better faced tomorrow in a refreshed hormonal state. Everything feels better after a good night's sleep!

Not All Pain Goes Away

Now that you understand sensation gating and have an idea of the complex role emotions and hormones play in your pain experience, it's time to re-examine chronic pain that doesn't seem to improve.

Remember that Plan B is the cheap, long-term fallback strategy that your body turns to when Plan A is repeatedly failing to complete. If the Plan B program can eventually finish, then the pain should go away, even if it has been going on for years. There is hope!

However, there are instances when your body has completed its repair plan but *there is still pain*. The war ended but no one told the infantry to come home. If you are experiencing this, you are not alone. Sometimes creating the conditions for a repair cycle to complete is not enough to stop the pain sensation, as pain has an added layer of complexity. To understand why pain remains after an injury has repaired, and what to do about it, we need to think more about emotions and hormones.

Chapter 18

EMOTIONS AND PAIN

To get a full picture of chronic pain, it's important to explore the role of emotions. Before we start, I want to make it clear that the relationship between emotions, memories, and pain is still a bit of a mystery. At this stage in our scientific knowledge, we understand that factors like emotions, beliefs, and past experiences play a significant and complex role in how we experience and respond to pain, as well as how we see the world, and that your experience is unique to you. Despite how sticky it is, this topic is one that I want to explore to the best of my ability. I hope this chapter will help you understand how your emotions and memories may be impacting your ongoing pain, preventing you from making the changes you want.

How Do You Feel Today?

Emotions are the feelings that tell you about the overall state of your body. The current state of your body depends on which of its "preset programs" are running. You may feel happiness, sadness, fear, pride, love, hate, envy, etc. Importantly, your emotions are changed by any factor that influences the overall state of your whole body.

How you feel is important. It is frustrating when someone tells you to stop feeling an emotion. Telling you to "cheer up – you have no reason to feel sad" does not work.

Your body is simply reporting on its hormonal state.

A lot of people struggle with how they feel because emotions can be difficult to understand. Everybody experiences them in a slightly different way.

Sensations are easier to compare. If I tell you to feel this hard, smooth table, we can both agree what hard and smooth feels like. We can both agree what a wet, slimy fish feels like. Emotions are more like the sensations of taste and smell. Try to describe what that fish smells or tastes like. A slightly nicer example is describing how your favourite chocolate bar tastes to your friend who has never had one. Once they taste it you can come closer to agreeing what it is like, but even then you will interpret the taste slightly differently.

Now, attempt to describe the emotion of happiness to your friend. This is much more difficult. Your emotions are complex, customized, hormonal states. We have no physical comparisons for emotions like we do with sensations. We can all feel happiness, but no one person's happiness is exactly the same as someone else's. This is why emotions can be so hard to understand. There is no standardized trigger for the happy emotion that we can all experience. Not everyone is ticklish or thinks my jokes are funny!

When you understand what an emotion is, you can start to learn why your body is telling you that you are happy, sad, tired, defeated, excited, anxious, or frustrated. Some people find it hard to admit that they feel a certain way when they don't see a logical reason for it. For example, admitting to yourself that you feel angry, even when you don't know why, is the first step to understanding this state for your body. Telling yourself that you shouldn't feel angry is not helpful. You do not need to understand a feeling to acknowledge that it is important. Simply being aware of the emotion puts you in a better place to be able to work out why you are feeling this way, try to work out its trigger, and potentially change it.

Why Do You Feel Like This Today?

When *emotions persist for a long time*, for instance, when you consistently feel sadness, you may feel like you are in a certain mood. An emotion is usually directly related to a recent event. It reports how your body responds to that event. The reason you are in a certain mood can be harder to relate to what is currently happening to you. You may ask your teenager, "Why are you so grumpy today?" They grunt and walk off.

A sustained mood probably relates to a prolonged hormonal state. Prolonged stress can lead to feelings of sadness and defeat, and decrease the threshold for anger and fatigue. People who are chronically sick or overworked are generally more prone to depression. Because your body is efficient, it adapts to this new prolonged state.

Think back to the shoe factory. Imagine it is now in war time. It is experiencing a decrease in demand for its hi-top sneakers and a massive drop in sales. Hobnail army boots are now in high demand. When this happens, the factory manager changes the production line from sneakers to army boots. In a similar way, if your body finds itself in a consistent state, it will adapt to that situation even if it is not desirable, such as a prolonged low mood. The resultant new operational state becomes depression.

Sometimes, however, your mood can feel unpredictable and not related to your circumstances, for example, you are on holiday but you still feel grumpy. Why is this?

There is something else going on in your body. As it is a self-regulating machine, not all hormones relate directly to your current situation. Hormones are also used to control automatic body functions. A change in the hormonal state may still be reported to you by how you feel (emotions).

An example of this is the significant fluctuation of hormones in menstruation, these monthly fluctuations can lead to a change in certain emotions. Pregnancy is also a time of rapid hormonal changes which can cause substantial, sometimes unpredictable, variation in emotions.

Teenagers can be all over the place. As they grow, they are flooded with emotions as their body's hormones instruct growth and development. If you have a grumpy teenager, it is highly likely that the problem they are having is that they do not understand why they feel this way. If they are growing, their high levels of changing hormones can cause massive emotional swings. Their anger, sadness, and exhaustion may be nothing to do with what's going on around them. Combine this with the large amount of energy required to grow and you can get an emotionally fragile and constantly irritated kid.

You don't understand your teenager because they have no ****ing clue why they feel this way today.

Hopefully now *you* do.

If life is going well and you are in an optimistic mood, you are more prone to positive emotions and less affected by negative emotions and sensations. Happier people are more likely to move past negative experiences and bounce back from a rush of hormones that produce anger or sadness. Optimism is synonymous with hope. If you are in a sustained pessimistic mood, then the opposite is true. Pessimism is synonymous with despair. These examples, like all emotions and moods, are modulated by underlying hormonal states.

Blending Hormones Creates an Emotional Palette

Your body is controlled by the neuro-endocrine system. This is a collection of nerves and hormones that work together to control your body's preset programs. For simplicity, we will talk about this system as if it only uses hormones. Your body reports the combination of hormones that are active, moment by moment, by giving you an emotional feeling.

In the last chapter, I introduced the concept that emotions are like paint colours (pleasure or love as white and anger as black). An emotion is a combination of different hormones. If emotions are paint colours, imagine that hormones are a vast array of paint pigments. Combining the hormonal pigments creates a uniquely blended emotional "colour" that you feel. If you look at a colour wheel, it is made up of all the different combinations of pigments. If you imagine combining your hormones in this way, they form an "emotions wheel." What colours are assigned to each emotion is up for debate. There are many varied examples of emotion colour wheels on the internet. Your hormones blend together in ways that are unique to you.

I first realized this when one of my colleagues complained that she was "hangry." She had been working all night and things had not gone as planned.

"What do you mean, hangry?" I asked.

"I'm hungry and angry. Hangry," she replied.

I offered up my lunch. "Fancy a carrot stick?"
"**** off!" she snapped, as she marched off down the corridor on the hunt for a more sugary alternative.

If you want, you can play a fun game of combining two emotions. Sleepy and happy can be blended to become "shlappy." Your amped-up, cliff-jumping friend is "frightcited" (frightened and excited) right before the plunge. Maybe it's safer just to watch a horror movie.

Your body learns to run programs to meet the demands of different situations. These programs are put into action by your body releasing hormones. The different hormones (pigments) are blended in varying quantities and create the emotion (colour of the paint). Your emotions report how your body is blending these different hormones. How your body does this is learned and changes throughout your life and is therefore unique to you.

This blending of hormones means that your emotions are not uniform, they are variable. If blue is sadness, you might be feeling deep indigo or you might be feeling turquoise depending on the combination of hormone "pigments" present. You are never purely angry or happy. You can feel complicated emotions, like excitement with a thrill of fear when you go skydiving, or both delight and sadness when you see a funny photo at a funeral.

Remember, just as with any colour, some emotions can become dominant over others, just as mixing black or white paint in with other colours can modify and eventually dominate them in high enough quantities.

Can You Change How You Feel?

As the demands on your body can change quickly so does its production of hormones. Hormones and their effects can be very short lived, sometimes minutes or less! Because emotions are connected to hormones, they also can be fleeting.

For instance, if you are cut off in traffic by a speeding driver, you will feel anger that lasts for as long as you maintain this hormonal state in your body. Your anger may fade away once you arrive at work and are distracted by the day ahead. However, you can reduce your anger sooner by purposefully changing your hormonal state. If you turn on an upbeat song that you love and sing along to it, you'll find that your anger dissipates almost immediately. However, if you turn on a thrash metal song you may become a raging monster!

Hormonal states can also be maintained for a long time. If you stay in a situation long enough, maintaining a hormonal state, your body adapts, and this is reported as a sustained emotion, or a mood. As an example, cortisol is the stress hormone that makes you feel angry. The longer you stay in a situation that makes you feel angry, the angrier you become. In this case, cortisol continues to be produced and builds up. It's kind of like tuning into your favourite narcissistic rap all day long or adding fuel to a fire that is already burning.

That same traffic incident could cause a surge of anger that you then hold towards all other drivers. If you dwell on this incident for the rest of your ride, tell your colleagues about it all day, play it over and over in your mind, and then tell your partner about it when you get home that evening, your anger is sustained and can become a mood. If you feel this way every day in traffic, you can become a rather angry person in general. People will start to notice and may call you *Kuppuswamy* (Indian origin meaning "lord of anger") if they are being nice or *vicious* &$@*#%^ if they are not.

The next time that something triggers anger in you, a good recommendation is to remove yourself from the situation and allow time for the hormone to wear off. Take deep, calming breaths. Your mother may have taught you to leave the room and count to ten, which is very wise. Watch something that will make you laugh. You will be amazed how quickly your anger dissipates. When you return to the situation, you can deal with it from a different hormonal state and create a better outcome. People will notice and may change your name from *Jerk to Joy*.

What Happens If You Can't Run Away?

In the previous chapter, I used the example of running away from a bear in the woods to talk about gating. This is an extreme example of when a stress response overrides other emotions and dampens sensations to get you out of a life-threatening situation. The truth is that most stress responses in the modern age are less about an immediate threat to life and more about long-term stress. However, our bodies still respond as if the situation is life threatening.

If your body is in an environment that you don't like, you feel a level of emotional "pain." Workplace stress is a common example of this. When you are in a situation like this, you experience a stress response that leads to *anxiety*. This form of emotional pain is felt as a response that urges you to leave the situation.

Adrenalin and cortisol are hormones that play a big part in this response. Adrenalin turns up the necessary machinery so that you are ready to run away. You may experience a high level of anxiety at this point or even have a panic attack. Once you move past the acute response, the adrenalin wears off, and you might feel a bit shaky.

Cortisol is a hormonal response that tells your body to release its readily available stored energy so that you have the fuel you need to fight or run away. It also does a neat trick and borrows energy from systems that you won't need while running away. One of these is your healing system. By turning off the healing it also turns off your pain response. You know that cortisol is in your system because your body reports this hormone by making you feel stressed out.

If you find your workplace stressful, this can start to have a lasting impact on both your mood and body, leaving you in a sustained state of anger, pessimism, anxiety, and fatigue. Your general mood is literally depressed.

Things get complicated when you cannot simply run away from the situation. While your stress response decreases right away when you escape from a bear, your most common stressors are likely not as simple. If you are not able to leave a stressful situation, or the situation is recurrent, like your job, your body will run its fight-or-flight response repetitively. If your surroundings do not change, or your hormonal response to those surroundings does not change, your stress and anxiety are reinforced and grow stronger.

Why Is Prolonged Stress Bad for You?

The threshold between tolerable and intolerable stress is not a choice you make. Especially in consistent, low-level stress environments, it's difficult to detect when a stress threshold has been passed because the environment is so normal for you. Unknown to you, a cortisol response is running all the time, and your general state of depression deepens.

This is where emotions, pain, and physical changes start to intertwine. For instance, if the cortisol response runs for too long, it may decrease your body's ability to repair and may increase wear and tear. Prolonged stress can lead to the craving of high-energy fuels that increase body weight. It can disturb sleep, increase fatigue, and lead to both escalating pain and failed healing attempts. As it becomes worse, your body can start to fail as it does not heal well. In extreme cases some consider ending their life to end the pain. Stress can literally kill you!

Why Do Some People Seem to Thrive on Stress?

Some people enjoy the feeling of stress when their flight-or-fight response and all their senses are heightened in the short term. They get very frightcited and may use the word "dude" a lot.

*"Wow, dude, this is sketchy. I'm not sure this is a good idea. Oh, **** it! Watch this..."*

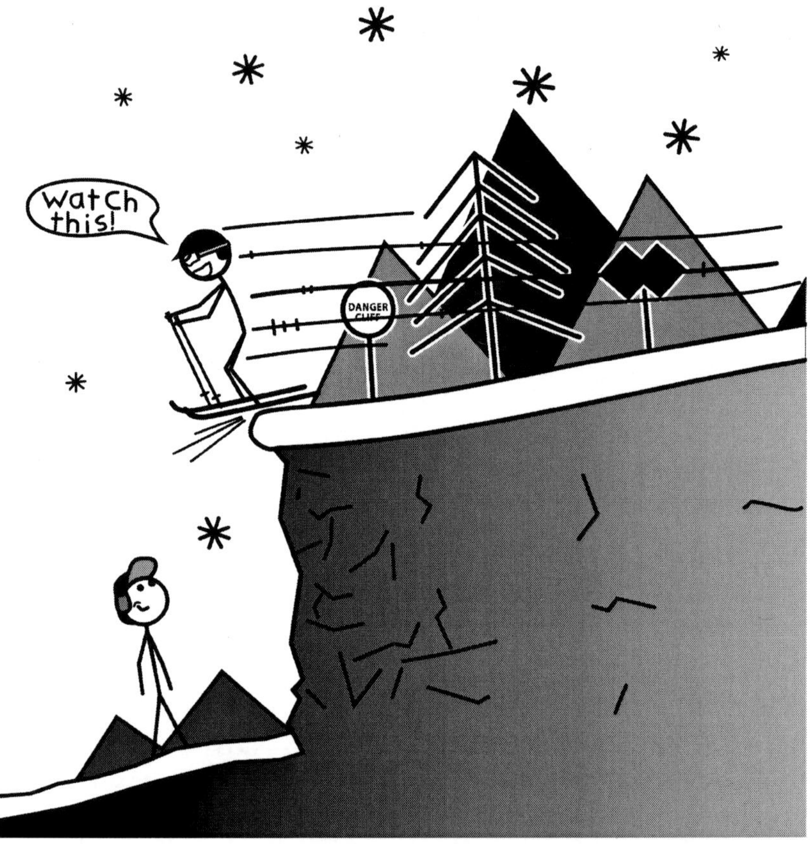

One of the benefits of being in this state is that your performance is increased by stress, up to a certain point. Athletes who do high-performance, high-intensity sport tend to enjoy a certain level of stress and try to increase it before they perform. People who enjoy this sensation also enjoy jobs where danger is a possibility and quick responses are important.

When your body is in a heightened state of stress, it is running as hard as it can. This can be pleasurable, as it leads to a buzzy feeling where you are hyperaware and can react more quickly than usual. However, not everybody wants the stress of being an athlete, surgeon, firefighter, or soldier. Not everyone wants to jump off cliffs or out of airplanes. It is all about control and consequences. Think about the difference between being an extreme skier blasting down a steep, double-diamond black slope and how you would feel doing it as a beginner skier with an infant strapped to your back!

As I've mentioned before, your hormonal responses reported as emotions are as unique as you are! This is part of why the role of emotions is so complex.

The Part that Emotions Play in Prolonging Pain

As you learned in Chapter 16, your body can learn to amplify pain. This means that if you have an injury and become focused on the pain, you begin to reinforce the pathways that tell you about that pain. When this happens, your body gets better at reporting on everything in the injured area and so you feel pain more easily. You can develop a "pain flywheel."

A good example of this is a whiplash injury caused by a motor vehicle accident. Whiplash happens when a car is hit from behind by another car, causing the front car's occupants to be forced back into their seats. If the head rest is not adjusted in a supportive position, this sudden movement can over-extend the neck, leading to muscle strain. A whiplash injury can take days to months to get over. Some people report ongoing pain for years.

We see that pain caused by a whiplash injury is often prolonged if a lawsuit is started. In these cases, the pain does not improve until litigation has finished, and the money is paid out. In many cases, this means that the pain continues even after the repair cycle has completed. What on earth does the legal process have to do with pain? We already know that the human body adapts to its circumstances and surroundings. This includes reporting pain. So, if you have a vested interest in pain, your body will report it better.

If you are suffering from whiplash, consider this: Every time you experience pain in your neck, it reminds you of the accident, and this brings up a lot of emotions. The pain reminds you that someone else is responsible for your injury. The anger, frustration, and exhaustion that comes from being in pain sets up a feedback loop that reinforces the pain connection.

In essence, your body gets better at reporting pain because you are training your brain to think about it. The unfortunate thing about this feedback loop is that it happens at an unconscious, automatic level. Very few people with whiplash injury decide to concentrate on their neck pain. The body does this on its own. The prevailing theory is that through a prolonged lawsuit process, which is a significant event in most people's lives, this feedback loop is constantly fed on an unconscious level. Once the process has completed, there are fewer reminders and the brain eventually ceases to have a vested interest in the event.

This phenomenon is very common and is sometimes called "sensitization" of a sensory response. It probably happens at the level of the spinal cord and is considered a problem in the pain reporting system. The "volume control" for this pain sensation has been turned up. It's as if the signal from the receptor is the same but amplified, like a volume control on your TV. Let's say most people watch their TV with the volume set at level six. But yours is stuck at ten and even the neighbours are complaining about the noise! It means that this pain is getting more attention than it normally would.

When enough time has passed that even the chronic inflammation program (Plan B) should have completed, something has gone wrong. This sensitization can be thought of as "Plan B+." The body has adapted to Plan B and continues in this state as the new normal. This is why some people rub their neck as they talk about a traffic collision from twenty years ago. Even though there is no longer an input to cause pain, the pain carries on. The war is over but for them it still continues.

A more emotional version of sensitization is post-traumatic stress disorder (PTSD). This is when something really bad has happened to you and you have ongoing flashbacks as you relive the event in your mind. The trigger for reliving this flashback can be the memory of the bad event or an emotion or sensation experienced during that event. How actions and behaviours are triggered is an important concept that we will save for later. What the treatment of PTSD has taught us is that every time you recall a memory you make it stronger. Therapists have found that repeatedly recalling a bad event makes the problem worse.

A problem shared is a problem halved.
A problem repeatedly shared is a problem multiplied!

The treatments for all of these chronic-pain conditions are very similar in that they help you reinterpret the memory and divert your painful thinking onto more positive things.

If you are experiencing chronic pain, there is always hope! With help you can learn to understand your pain, develop strategies to decrease its impact on your life, and function better with it. You can take control of your pain, rather than allowing it to control you. Your reporting system is very sensitive, so this is not always easy, but it is worth it. We will discuss this more in Chapter 30. First, let's get a better idea of how our emotions are involved in prolonging pain.

What Can You Do If You Can't Run Away?

You should probably try to get rid of the bear, but sometimes it just won't stay away! If you can't change the circumstances that are causing you stress and depression, you can manage the stress by diluting the stress hormones with other hormones. In other words, you can find ways to control how you feel, to create more reassurance, control, and optimism in your inner world until you can begin to change your outer world.

Some activities release hormones that *decrease* feelings of stress; these include exercise, spending time in the sunshine, being sociable with people you love, and doing fun activities that bring you a lot of satisfaction. For many people, getting a pet is life-changing when it comes to alleviating depression.

Pursuing activities like these give you a sense of control and choice in the matter and empower you to eventually change your external circumstances in a beneficial way. Importantly, in the same way that you can adapt any part of your body, you can adapt your hormonal systems to your circumstances. If you allow yourself to get angry regularly, you get better at it. If you do pleasurable activities, you get better at experiencing pleasure. Your body will adapt to whatever you do repeatedly. Later we will learn that this includes thinking about something a lot as well.

Meditation, breathing, and mindful exercises also help with stress management. In moments of anger, sadness, fear, or anxiety, stop and remove yourself from the situation. Use mindfulness or meditation to help bring awareness to your emotions, think about what has caused them and then allow the stress hormones to dissipate.

Stop, think, breathe.

A good technique lots of people use is breathing deeply and slowly (some use counting in their heads to help slow breathing down, e.g., breathe in, two, three, four; hold, two, three, four; breathe out, two, three four ...). This tells your body to stop running the fight-or-flight "anxiety program" and change to the "relaxed and thoughtful" program. Breathing into a paper bag is a good, old trick that causes the respiratory system to slow down its rate when you are panicking. Within a few minutes, your body will return to its regular operational mode.

Busting a Chronic Pain Myth

There is a misleading story about chronic pain that has done a lot of damage in our world. The story is that *chronic pain is imagined* or "in your head." If you have heard this, or believe it on some level, I hope that with the knowledge I have shared, we can collectively put this myth to rest.

Pain is not purely mechanical, which means that it cannot be solved only through mechanical strategies like surgery or exercises.

The truth is that all pain is real, and all pain has an emotional element to it; one that we are still learning about. This means that while you can work on helping your body to heal, it's just as important to examine other factors that may be contributing to and prolonging your pain. *Every body hurts* in a personalised way.

If this resonates with you, remember that emotional pain is generally felt when there is a loss of control of your situation.

One of the best things you can do for your chronic pain is to seek mental health support.

Addressing your emotional pain and the circumstances that prolong it will help you manage your physical pain.

PART 4

The Capacity Game

Chapter 19

MEDICATION'S ROLE IN PAIN MANAGEMENT

Your body has the capacity to repair and, as we have discussed, it can be exceeded. It is ultimately your body that repairs itself, but sometimes it needs outside help, especially when you find yourself in a "no fix" situation. This help can include physical therapy, surgery, medications, or a combination of these strategies.

Sometimes your body has gone far enough over capacity that the resulting injury is just too painful to stand. Your body may be trying so hard to fix you that it exceeds your capacity to tolerate the pain associated with that fix. The older I get, the more I realize you can't always fix everything on your own.

In this chapter, we will talk briefly about medications: How they work, what their role is, and how they are used effectively, because when they are not used effectively, they create more problems. By the end, you should feel better equipped to decide when medication is a good option for you.

Medications and drugs can be considered anything you put into your body that alters how its systems function.

Generally, medications are absorbed through a mucous membrane (such as your gut or lungs) or your skin and are distributed throughout the body by your bloodstream.

Anything you put in or on your body, whether it's food, pills, supplements, or creams, affects how your body runs. Doctors tend to talk about "medications" when they are prescribed and "drugs" when there is a negative connotation. For example, if a doctor prescribes a narcotic pain killer, it is considered a medication. However, if you became addicted to that pain pill, the same doctor might say you have a "drug addiction." Others simply call them pills. Regardless of what language is used, their purpose is to create a change in the body.

How Do Medications Work?

Medications are used to help the body do something it is currently not doing. Generally, they do one of the following:

1. Supply, replace, or maintain a raw material or hormone that your body is deficient in or has stopped producing enough of. An example is taking vitamin C to treat scurvy or the hormone thyroxine if your thyroid is not working properly. Another example is taking an anti-depressant that artificially elevates levels of "happy hormones" like serotonin.

2. Interfere with a process in the body. An example of this is an antibiotic, which helps fight off an unwanted bacteria invader. The antibiotic poisons the bacteria and they stop replicating or die. The antibiotic may also cause some collateral damage to you, but it helps you win the battle against the bug. You could liken it to throwing a hand grenade when you're in a gun fight.

3. Instruct a system to run or to work in a different way. An example of this is taking a medication for diabetes to make your sugar metabolism work harder. Another example is taking a sleeping pill to help you fall asleep. Pain pills also fall into this category. Pain pills tell your body not to report the pain signal. Anti-inflammatories are medications that turn down the pain by turning down healing.

Medications are great rescuers but poor facilitators.

Take sleeping pills, for instance. If you can't sleep, it may be better to take a pill and sleep than not sleep at all. However, it's better to try everything else first. The best sleep you can get is regular, unmedicated sleep, and no pill can give you that. With medications it's good to ask yourself: Is this truly a rescue situation or is there another way to try first? Sometimes medications are just being used as an easy fix.

Functionally, medications are quite simple, but their effects are highly complex. They lack the subtlety of the finely tuned control that your body has developed. A signal that shouts "Stop healing!" obviously does not just affect the thing that is causing you pain. It affects the whole of your body.

Think of a medication as a "manual override button" on a space rocket. When there is a malfunction in one of its automatic systems and warning lights are shining on the overhead console, this override button lets the pilot manually take over everything. Just like that button, a medication tells your body: "Just ***ing do it!"

Medications cause many effects based on what they do.

We call desirable effects "therapeutic effects," and undesirable effects "side effects." A good rule of thumb is that a medication is useful if it's helping you more than it's hurting you. This is a fine balance, and the medication dose is important. Too little may do nothing helpful and too much may cause mayhem.

Important Things to Consider When Taking a Medication

Before we learn about some different types of medications and how they manage pain and discomfort, there are four important things to understand:

1. Generally, any medication that influences your body will cause adaptation. This means that if you use a medication regularly, it will lead to some level of dependence, as well as symptoms of withdrawal when you stop taking it. The consequences of becoming dependent on a medication are related to what it is doing to your body and the dosage you are taking. Dependence can be a very bad thing, as in cases of alcohol or street-drug addiction. However, it is not always a bad thing, like in the example of thyroxine, which keeps you alive when your thyroid has stopped working.

2. All medications have adverse side effects. Manipulating your body into solving one problem is not possible without creating a different problem. Think of a medication infomercial where the list of side effects is longer than the list of benefits! In some cases, experiencing new issues because of a medication is worth it, such as when that medication is lifesaving or life-sustaining. However, many people end up taking a cocktail of medications to handle the side effects created by their initial medications. Again, the dose of the medication is also an important factor here, as most side effects increase with an increased dose.

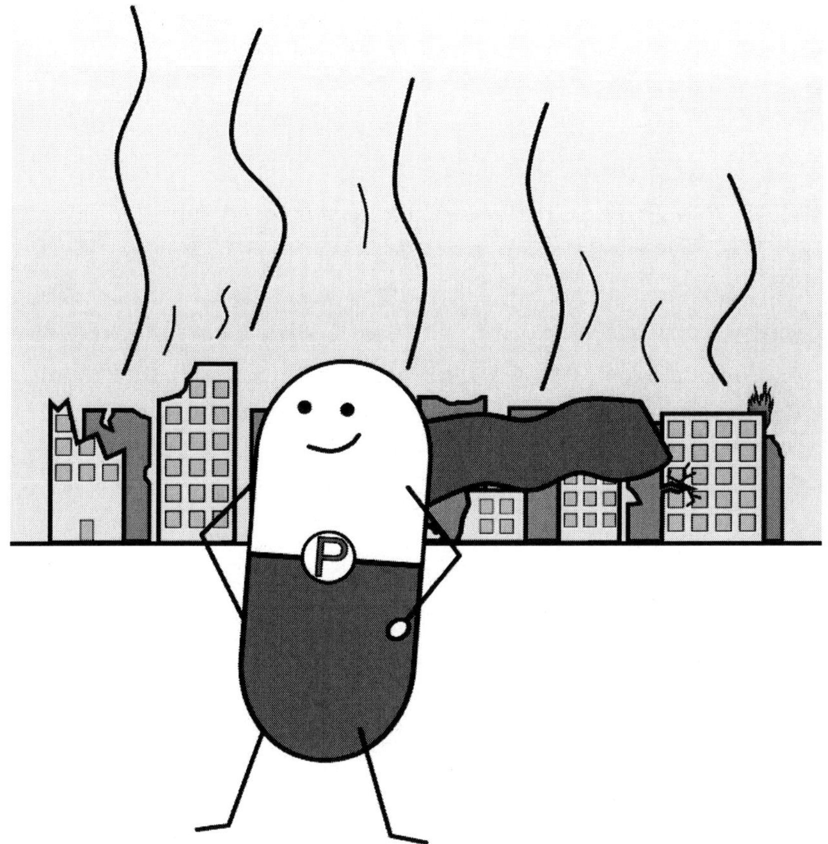

Captain Pill** and the attack of the **Nasty Infectants** includes **collateral damage!

3. Medications are not magic. Medications are used to interfere with metabolic processes. If you are in pain, a pill that messes with your pain pathways can change your experience of pain or stop you from feeling the pain for a while. This is desirable if your pain is preventing you from functioning.

However, it's important to remember that there is no such thing as a drug that stops you feeling your pain without consequences. A pain killer affects everything it meets. It may reduce your headache, but it also impacts all other systems in your body. Medications are hard on your systems. Therefore, it is important to be thoughtful when taking any medication.

4. Medications are not as good as the "real thing." Sleeping with a pill is not as good quality as without. You heal faster without an anti-inflammatory (more on that to follow). Your body works better if you don't take the antibiotic. Your recovery from depression is better without the medication. Exercise is better than the high blood pressure pill. Remember what I said at the beginning of the chapter, though, sometimes you just can't do it on your own. If you could, there would be no doctors and no need for this book.

Before You Opt for Medication

Medications can be, and often are, taken as an easy fix. If you have a headache, the simplest solution is to take a pain killer. If you become diabetic, it's easier for your doctor to prescribe a medication that makes your already failing digestive system work harder, rather than assist you in changing your habits as a form of treatment. This is largely the cultural and social result of wanting to *feel better quickly and effortlessly*.

When taken as an easy fix, a medication can allow the continuation of behaviours that are damaging to your body.

You could say that in some circumstances medications are *permissive* – they allow you to carry on when you would be better off making a change. If your knees hurt, for example, you can take medication that dampens the pain so you can keep playing soccer. Meanwhile, your knees are sending you pain signals to *stop* you from playing, because doing so is increasing the amount of damage that will need to be fixed. When you take pain medication in this way, it's like putting in earplugs so you can ignore what your body is saying.

Although problematic, prescribing medications for pain and discomfort is often easier for both patient and doctor and is also very profitable for the companies making these medications. We must remember that it is truly not in the interest of drug companies to make us healthy again.

So, let's consider other ways you can address your symptoms before turning to medication. As I mentioned earlier, medication can include anything you put into your body that alters its systems' functions, so this includes food! When food is digested, some of its parts can act as hormone signals changing how you feel. Eating the right food provides the fuel and raw materials you need to run your systems. When things go wrong, a good place to start is ensuring your body is receiving the best food for its situation. Eating the right food can help you feel better and heal as fast as possible, which ultimately decreases your pain.

The right food differs between bodies and circumstances. For example, if you have a flu and you're fifty years old, you'll need different food than a thirty-year-old training for a marathon in a month. If you have digestive system damage due to an infection, it may be better to rest your gut and rely on fluids and fuel reserves until your guts have won their battle and repaired themselves. Before heading to the pharmacy, consider how changing what you eat and drink may help.

If you consider food as a form of medication, you will realize that it also has good effects and bad effects. Food contains what you need but can be packaged with things that may harm you. A good rule of thumb is:

Healthy food gives you what you need at the time whilst doing the least amount of damage.

Generally, the least damaging food is the least processed food. It's important to note that there are no universal superfoods. A superfood is simply a food that contains something that your body is lacking or needs to function normally.

Pain Medications

Your body uses pain signals to tell you that you are hurt, and these signals stay on to remind you that you are under repair. The job of pain medications is to make this pain tolerable or go away completely. Depending on the medication, it modulates the pain reporting system either at the pain receptor or in the nerves. When you think about pain medications, most people think of narcotics, such as codeine and morphine, which work by blocking the pain receptors.

Acetaminophen is one of the most commonly used pain killers. Interestingly, it is not known exactly how it works, but it is probably by blocking prostaglandins in the brain. Prostaglandins have many functions and one is involved in the control of pain signal transmission. Blocking prostaglandins seem to help reduce the transmission of pain signals in the brain. It also can reduce fevers. It does not seem to directly affect inflammation.

Another common type of pain medication blocks the inflammatory pathways. We have already met the hormone cortisol in fight-or- flight and stress responses. Cortisol is also manufactured by drug companies to be used as a medication. This "steroid" anti-inflammatory hormone medication is used when you need to turn down your body's pain by turning down its healing. More on cortisol in the next section.

Another class of medication that turns down inflammation is *not a steroid hormone*. Imaginatively, these medications are called "not cortisone" or non-steroidal anti-inflammatories (NSAIDs), the best known one is ibuprofen. NSAIDs are very commonly used for pain, especially in musculoskeletal injuries.

Consider how an anti-inflammatory medication is anti-healing. By reducing inflammation to relieve pain, the medication turns down the healing process. As with all medications, this doesn't mean that anti-inflammatories are all bad (in fact, they are very necessary and helpful in certain circumstances); however, slowing down the healing process plus masking pain puts you at risk of more damage.

There are other types of pain medications for special uses. These modulate nerves in the peripheral nervous system and the brain. Local anesthetics, such as those injected by the dentist, are the best known for blocking peripheral nerves. Chemical signals in the pain reporting system can also be modulated; for example, anti-depressants are used to modulate pain by increasing happy hormones in the brain. Other medications can change how nerve signals are transmitted. Messing with your pain-reporting machinery can make your experience of pain more tolerable.

Can Taking Pain Killers Make Things Worse?

We've not had a machine story for a while, so humour me! Imagine one day your pickup truck starts to overheat and the check engine light comes on. You take it to the mechanic who tells you that, no surprises, the truck needs fixing. However, you need to use the truck that day, so he reluctantly agrees that you can come back another day. He puts a sticker over the temperature gauge and check engine light to stop them from distracting you.

"It's not fixed," he tells you, "but if you go easy on it, you should be okay. Don't worry about that gauge and light for now. We'll get the truck fixed when you have time." Things go okay for a while. *Maybe the truck doesn't need fixing after all*, you think. Since it seems fine, you decide to ignore the mechanic and tow a trailer with it. Not long into your journey, you find yourself on the side of the road with steam pouring from the engine. You go back to the mechanic. "I told you not to overdo it until I fixed it!" he protests. "Now you'll need a bigger fix." He books the truck for some "engine surgery."

Pain pills act like that sticker on the gauge and light. It's nice to not feel the pain, but it doesn't mean you're fixed – you're just not getting the message. It's worse than this though because an anti-inflammatory pill turns down your pain *by turning down your ability to heal*. This can make it easier to push yourself harder than you should and means you will heal even more slowly. Taking NSAIDs or pain pills makes it more likely that you will push your body into Plan B.

If you hit your thumb with a hammer and still have a painful thumb the next day, the smartest thing to do is not hit it again! Who would take a pain pill so they could hit their injured thumb again? What we tend to do is take a pill to "hack the system." People say, "I don't have time to heal, I'm far too busy."

Common examples include taking a pain pill so you can play soccer when you are injured, "My team is relying on me"; or so you can walk up a mountain again with your arthritic knee when you overdid it the day before, "We were on holiday and it was such a beautiful day!" This hacking the system is a common misuse of pain medication. We cover up the pain with a sticker, overdo it, and then wonder why the pain is much worse when the pain killer wears off! Holidays are a common cause of tipping people with arthritis into Plan B!

This may be a good time to consider why the steroid cortisone has gained a dubious reputation. A very common use of cortisone is in Plan B situations, when it is injected into joints or around tendons, to try to stop a healing process that is too painful or seems to have failed as it has gone on too long. Cortisone is injected as crystals that slowly dissolve and therefore have an extended hormonal effect lasting two weeks. Cortisone seems to turn off acute inflammation (Plan A) and chronic inflammation (Plan B). This "reboot" combined with "relative rest" can be enough to kick the injured part back into plan A. This can be a good thing, if you can then stay in Plan A. The reboot can keep the pain under control for a long time.

If cortisone is not used correctly, it can make things worse. If in the two weeks after an injection, you think the steroid has fixed you, and you overdo it while your pain and healing are turned off, you may regret it. In the 1960s cortisone injections were commonly used in sport to help injured soccer players continue to play. They were not even in Plan B, they just wanted to get back to playing quicker. They "did not have time to heal"! This trick quickly wore off in a week or two and, as they had been playing on an injury, the player inevitably then felt worse, prompting more cortisone injections. This worked a few times but with an escalating injury the player was so much worse off that eventually the pain stopped going away. The end of their careers was quickly associated with steroid use. Obviously turning off pain and healing can be a bad idea.

When Does Turning Down Pain Help Me?

Pain pills play an important role when pain becomes unbearable. When you are very injured or sick, pain dramatically reduces your function. It is generally better to heal without pills, but sometimes the pain becomes too much when your body is working hard to fix something. Think about the pain of breaking a bone or how your body aches when you get a flu virus.

No one likes being in pain. Pain is ****ing painful! There are no prizes for being in pain.

At times like these, it's important to find a balance between experiencing less pain and prolonging your repair time, risking Plan B. Always consider whether you are opting for a pain killer for rescue or facilitation. For instance, after a surgery, an NSAID is often prescribed to rescue you from the pain due to the major overload injury and the amount of inflammation that is required to fix it. Consider other types of pain pills first, such as acetaminophen. If your pain becomes "sweary bad," talk to your doctor about whether something stronger is appropriate in the short term. If you take an NSAID it can feel like magic in the short term, but it may also slow healing and prolong the injury.

Pain pills are sometimes the lesser of two evils. They can be a great option if your pain is preventing you from sleep, which is so important for repair. We all need to be rescued sometimes! It may be better to take a pill, for a short time, when you are recovering from an injury, illness, or surgery, than to not sleep at all. Sometimes your body "malfunctions" and NSAIDs can be used as a kind of reset button. Migraines and muscle spasms are examples of this. Taking the pill should still be reserved for rescue in order to reboot the system, if the usual things like rest and fluids for a migraine, or getting a massage for muscle spasms, don't help. In some circumstances a short course of anti-inflammatories may be used to try to reboot an injury that has gone into plan B. This may involve taking ibuprofen for a limited time (two to fourteen days) or having a cortisone injection. As we already discussed, this is for rescue only and should be used with care, usually under the supervision of a medical professional.

For lesser pain, it is better to use other strategies, starting with listening to what your pain is telling you. Focus on maximizing your healing factors (such as not smoking, healthy foods, sleep etc.). You can heal faster by avoiding more overload and allowing for adequate repair time. Getting enough rest is a big factor in all of this. Allowing repair to complete is the best way to shut down the pain. For a big injury or repair, unfortunately this can take weeks or months. In a gun fight, it is nice to have a fallback plan. When you are in pain it is good to have medications to rescue you when things get too much. In a gun fight, sometimes you just need a hand grenade!

A Powerful Mindset

When it comes to healing and pain management, I find a person's *attitude* is the biggest predictor of how well they will do with treatments. Sometimes people just want to *feel* better now; they simply do not want to feel pain anymore. They are often wanting an easy fix to their long-standing problems. Sometimes they have been like this for so long and have adapted to this new normal so well that they may have lost the hope of ever getting better. At this stage, they are in chronic pain (Plan B+). They can appear to not want to get better. This is generally not a conscious decision they have made, but rather due to the feeling that they have lost control of their body. If you are experiencing this, it is essential to remember that there is always hope:

It doesn't matter how long your body has been broken, your body still wants to make you better.

You need to work with your body, not against it. People who do want to get better give their body's repair system permission to work. They do not rely on medications as a *sole* treatment or solution and instead look for other ways to support their repair, seeking assistance from physical therapists, dieticians, mental health professionals, and other tools available. The decision to allow repair is the most essential part of this process.

You are in charge.
You must give your body permission to heal.

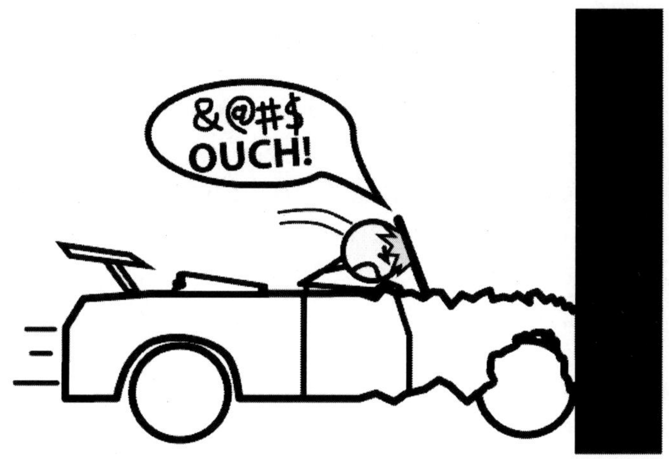

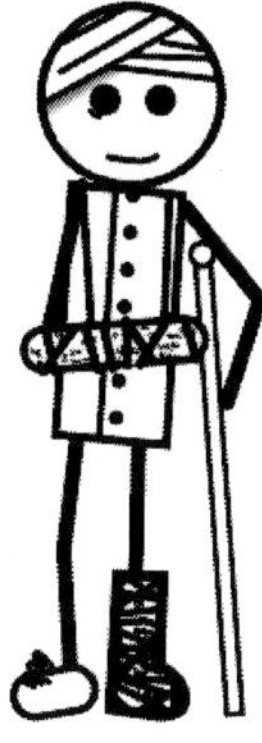

**Hey body,
that ****ing hurt but I know
you've got this and will do
your best to fix me up!
Take the time you need.
Let me know what you want
me to do!**

Chapter 20

DECONDITIONING

This is how a typical story goes: A former marathon runner has experienced pain in her right knee for about ten years. The source of her pain is not a mystery; for her adolescence and much of her adult life, she ran consistently and trained for long distances. Her right knee has a minor, long-forgotten, decades-old injury and so it started to wear out quicker than the left. Nothing dramatic happened, she simply got older.

She started to experience increased overload pain from her runs. The pain started out minimally, so she ran through it. Then it started to ache more, so she rubbed her knee to make it feel better between runs. Eventually, it hurt whether she was running or not. Walking, or even just sleeping in a certain position, started to cause pain. She was entering the Plan B chronic inflammation repair program. She decided to stop running, but the pain persisted. However, as time went on, the pain decreased slowly and one day she realized ... *it was gone.*

How did this happen? The concept is simple. If you reduce the load on an overloaded system (in this case, by stopping running), the chronic inflammation repair cycle will eventually finish. Plan B completes its economical rescue program. This explains how chronic overload injuries eventually get better over time without particular effort. To return to the war metaphor, it's as if the infantry is called home after many months of inaction on the battlefield. However, the battlefield left behind is not a pretty sight, with lots of unfinished projects and messy debris littered about. It could be a beautiful place again, but for now it is a wasteland and is being ignored. Deconditioning has set in.

Why Can't I Do What I Used To?

The runner's pain has gone away because she stopped running, but there are consequences to not using her knee normally. When she stopped running, she also stopped doing other things that caused her discomfort, like hiking, going for walks in the evening, and taking the stairs at work. It's likely she didn't even notice the ways she adapted her movements over time to avoid pain. However, it now means that her knee has deconditioned with a reduced capacity and can be easily overloaded. She can no longer do what she used to. As we touched on in the emotions chapter, there is another layer here; this injury has caused her a lot of frustration, fear, and depression related to how she felt when she chose to stop doing the thing she loved: running.

Many people who experience a growing, nagging injury reach a fork in the road – they can either stop doing what they love or get professional help to address it. Perhaps you have been at this fork before. The first road means giving up and allowing part of your body to decondition. This deconditioning results in loss of muscle tone and overall fitness. You may also walk or move in a funny way to adapt to the injury. For our runner, it means choosing to use her knee less for the rest of her life. For someone who loves running, this is a big deal. The second road means facing up to the problem and seeking help. For some fiercely independent people, acknowledging they need help can also be a big deal!

There are things other than injuries that can put us "out of action" as well. Any illness can put you in bed or limit your activities. Even a nasty cold or flu bug virus like COVID-19 that attacks your whole body can put you out of action long enough to significantly decondition.

Astronauts in Space

When I meet a patient for the first time, I look for a "key" to unlock their presenting problem. The key is what I call a deconditioning event. Why is deconditioning such an important piece in the puzzle? Just like our runner, if you stop doing something, your body down-regulates very quickly. Although we'll all experience some form of deconditioning, astronauts provide a good illustration of the rule:

Use it or lose it!

Let's board a space rocket and escape the loading effect of gravity on our bodies. Astronauts spend a significant amount of time floating without any load on their muscles and bones at all. Over days and weeks in space, an astronaut's muscles and bones adapt to the lower loads. In this sense, the lack of gravity acts like a disease, causing decreased capacity in the musculoskeletal system through lack of work. The Space Station has resistance exercise equipment on board to help astronauts avoid extreme deconditioning. While resistance exercises are very important for astronauts, they still decondition; there is no replacement for the constant load of gravity.

When an astronaut returns to Earth, gravity makes them "heavier" again and increases the load on their body. By this time, their body has adapted to the lower demands of space. Imagine having to face this sudden increase in demand! Because of this, returning astronauts are very weak, sometimes unable to stand up against the force of gravity. If they have been in space for a long time they can be as weak as a newborn baby, unable to even lift their head! The good news is that this initial weakness upon returning to Earth is short-lived. Astronauts recover quickly because they can't escape gravity and therefore can't avoid doing work. Here's another way to think about it:

If lack of gravity acts likes a disease, the only treatment for an astronaut is to add gravity back into their life!

Simply being back on Earth for an astronaut is like a full-body workout all day long. The body quickly "remembers" what it used to do. For every day they spend in space, it takes about a day to recover.

However, things get much worse if the astronaut is in space for a very long time indeed. Sometimes an astronaut's body systems never fully recover from the decreased load and disuse they experience in space. The longer an astronaut spends in space, the larger the "overload injury of weightlessness." They start to lose minerals from their bones, something that cannot be fully repaired when they come back to Earth. In these cases, their bones will never be quite as strong again. Their time in space can be considered a "catastrophic deconditioning event."

Although this is an extreme example of whole-body deconditioning that the average person won't experience, we can apply the same principles to us. In the running example, the runner's knee becomes deconditioned through lack of use. Like an astronaut, you can regain capacity but if you lose enough capacity in a system, it may not fully regain its pre-injury capacity.

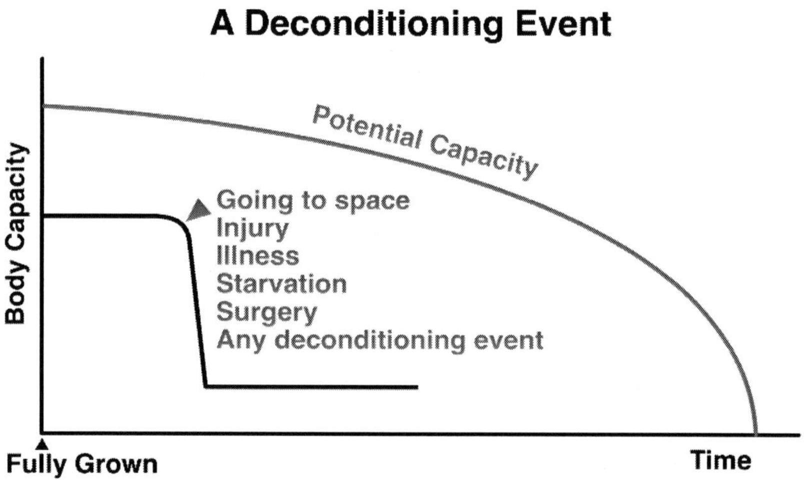

How Quickly Do You Decondition?

How quickly you decondition depends on where you are starting from. Remember the flywheel example with the two brothers? One brother has been training for a marathon much harder and for much longer than the other brother. If they both stop training on the exact same day, both their flywheels begin to run down but at different rates. The first brother's flywheel has a lot more momentum and runs for longer, which means it will take longer for him to decondition. The second brother's flywheel has a lot *less* momentum, which means that once he stops running, deconditioning sets in quickly. Similarly, if you have built up strong capacity in a system through continued training over many years, you will decondition more slowly after injury than someone who has trained less.

Another factor that affects deconditioning is how much you continue to use your injured system. If you completely stop doing an activity, like the two brothers who quit running, you lose your capacity more quickly than if you do some maintenance. Stopping an activity entirely increases your risk of an overload injury, while exercising even once a week can be enough to help maintain capacity and prevent deconditioning.

Astronauts who do resistance exercises in space decondition more slowly than those who do not. In the same way, if you continue to play an instrument or golf occasionally, you do not lose your skills as quickly as if you stopped altogether. This is a balancing act. Sometimes you must accept some deconditioning to allow repair to complete. We all tend to be impatient and try to get back to activities too quickly. Therefore, learning to listen to your body and do what it is telling you is so important.

The trick is to recognize if you have forced your body into Plan B. My best advice in this situation is to accept that this program has started and that it will take some extra time to finish. If you think you are in Plan B, this may be the time to seek some help. You don't have to wait for the Plan B program to finish completely before returning to activity, but you may need some help and advice to come up with a personalized strategy. You can slowly start to use Plan A to save the day!

This strategy even works if you're in Plan B+. We will discuss how to do this in the coming chapters.

Climbing Out of the Deconditioning Hole

Let's go back to the second road at the fork: seeking professional help. Rather than choosing to stop doing what you love to avoid pain, you can choose to regain function in your injured area. The good news is that you now have an advantage because of your knowledge about the tear and repair cycle. Like the astronaut, you can *recondition*.

If lack of movement acts likes a disease, the only treatment for deconditioning is to add movement back into your life!

After the "inciting event" that caused you to decondition is over, you can get better again. You may not be the same as before, but you must work with what you've got. You can even improve "chronic fatigue" if you work at it slowly, with *baby steps*. Remember the astronaut with the strength of a baby after a year in space! Reconditioning takes a heavy dose of patience and persistence. I must admit, your body can feel really "****ing annoying" during reconditioning, like it has given up on you. It hasn't.

In my own practice, I have been most successful with people who have chronic pain by encouraging them to *slowly* improve their capacity over time. Let's say you have a knee injury. If you stay within your knee's reduced load capacity, you will not experience more pain, but your knee will also weaken and decondition over time. However, if you incrementally increase load through completed training cycles (overload with complete repair), you can slowly increase the load that your knee can take without it becoming too overloaded and painful. I have watched this simple concept turn around people's injuries and lives with improved health outcomes as a result. The key is in understanding the importance of minor overload and repair, rather than trying for too much, too soon ... or not trying at all. It's about finding the middle ground. Chapter 30 is all about this.

Chapter 21

UNWANTED WEIGHT GAIN

At some point in our lives, we all find something that we would like to change. Ask any of your friends and they will offer endless advice on things that you could change (but only in a helpful, non-offensive, loving, you-are-just-fine-as-you-are–but-if-you-wanted-to–not-saying-that-you-have-to–only-if-it-is-really-important-to-you-and-your-life's-journey–possibly–maybe-without-being-critical–you-could kind of way). There is more to life than healing injuries and building bigger muscles. Can we use the principle of efficiency-guided change to understand other areas of our bodies?

One of the most common changes we observe over time is body weight and shape. In our modern world, unwanted body weight has, for some, become an obsession. The questions of why we gain more of it, and how to maintain a healthy weight effectively, have become a huge focus and continue to feed the billion-dollar-diet-and-exercise industry. As with all the topics I've covered in this book, my aim when I talk about unwanted weight gain (and believe me, I've been there) is to illustrate the principles behind it: why we gain unwanted weight, how the cycle of overload and repair applies, and the role of both food and hormones in weight change.

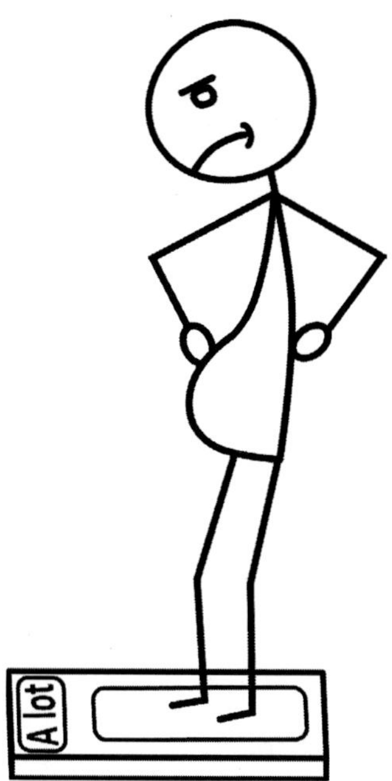

Why Do We Gain Weight?

When you were born, you were probably less than 10 lbs of total body weight. As you grew into a toddler, then a child, and then a teen, your weight increased as your size increased. You were growing! Once you finished growing into your adult size, different factors started playing a role in your weight.

If you focus on building muscle by adapting to heavier loads, you gain weight. However, if you stop going to the gym you lose muscle mass, and it turns to fat. Fat weighs less than muscle, so this is the easiest weight loss you can experience, but it's not ideal. This is because by "gaining weight," most of us mean gaining *fat*. So, a better question is: Why do we gain fat? It's all because of our old friend, efficiency.

When your body does anything, it tries to be the most economical it can be. In any state of overload, remember that your body cannot see the future. It does not understand your good intentions. It doesn't know about your New Year's resolutions. It doesn't understand that you're going mountain biking tomorrow for the first time in your life. As I've said before:

Your body doesn't understand what you want it to do, it only understands what you do.

You communicate with your body through your actions, and it gathers information from your past to respond in the present. This is an important concept to keep in mind when you consider weight gain.

Food, the Currency of Life

Food is a collection of resources that are digested by your body. During digestion, the food you eat is separated into things your body can use and things it cannot use. The usable parts of your food are kept for fuel or as raw materials. This fuel gives you the energy you need to run your systems. The raw materials are used to both build the machinery and make the things you need for those systems. This whole process, just like Plan A (quick repair), is very expensive in terms of time and energy, so your body makes the most of what it is given.

There is a limit to how much fuel your body can use in a day.

Just as your muscles have a maximum capacity, so does your whole body. How much your whole body can do is limited by the amount of energy that it can make available to run all its systems. To do work, your body literally burns the fuel you provide it. This fuel comes from either food you recently ate or from your fuel stores. In Chapter 12 ("Why Your Capacity Matters"), we talked about how burning fuel requires oxygen, which means that how much work your body can do in a day is limited by how much air you can move.

Fuel is crucial to your body. Just like a car, without fuel, you can't do anything. Knowing how expensive it is for your body to digest food, you can start to understand how efficiency plays a role in this whole process. Digesting your food involves a lot of work: sorting the resources in food into fuel and raw materials. However, food can also contain bad things that damage your body. Your food may contain preservatives, colourings, pesticides, flavour enhancers, thickeners, microplastics, harmful bacteria and even medications (steroids, antibiotics, pain killers etc.). Your body has to selectively pick through all the good and bad ingredients, then repair any damage caused in the process. Eating hotdogs could be considered an extreme sport!

Your digestive system processes your food and tries to store whatever you don't need for immediate use. Storing resources is far more efficient than wasting them. After all, since your body cannot tell the future, it doesn't know if more food is coming. It is still convinced the apocalypse is around the corner or that one day the grocery store will run out of food. Your body is concerned with keeping you alive and functional for as long as it can.

For most raw materials there is an upper limit to how much can be stored, before it is more efficient to get rid of it. Your body has to get rid of even useful things because too much of anything can cause damage. For this reason, if you have a normal diet, most of the content of your expensive daily vitamin pill goes down the toilet to avoid overload damage. If a toddler gets into your medicine cabinet and eats your iron pills as candy, it can be fatal. We all know that dehydration can kill you but drinking too much water can overload your "water management machinery" causing your blood to become dilute and your brain to swell enough to finish you off as well. Too much water can be bad for you on the inside as well as the outside.

As you may have guessed, this efficient system can have consequences that add up over time. Say you eat a *lot* of food one day as you can't resist the two for one deal at the local pizza place. By eating too much food, not only do you risk giving your digestive system too much work to do resulting in a belly ache, you have also overloaded your energy (fuel) needs for that day. In principle this is the same as overloading your muscles at the gym. Just as a muscle upgrade means your muscles get bigger, eating too much food prompts your body to upgrade storage capacity so that the energy is available for another day. Both can result in your body getting bigger and heavier!

The excess energy is stored as fat, which allows your body to keep it locked away for a "rainy day" when there is not enough fuel around. As energy means life, energy stores are treated with the utmost importance. If doomsday never comes, those reserves are never used. If this habit becomes consistent, if you consume more energy in the form of food than is burned, then your body will continue upgrading its capacity for storage. Your body treats storing fat like building up a bank account. With lots of fat stored it is content because it has "loadsamoney"! There seems to be no upper limit to how big your body thinks that bank account should be. This can be very frustrating if you don't want to gain fat stores, but it's just your body being efficient. This was a huge realization for me when I tried to lose a few pounds. Stay tuned for that story in Part 5!

While fat stores will help you survive if there is no food around, they do have a cost. You not only have to carry those fat stores around with you but must maintain them as well. This is expensive for your body. We will consider the consequences of this later in Chapter 23 ("Exceeding Your Body's Capacity") when we talk about giving the body too much to do.

So, if you feel like your bank account is bulging, how do you persuade your body to spend its precious fat stores or rainy-day fund?

What about Going to a Bootcamp?

Bootcamps, which utilise exercise and altered eating habits, are a popular method for trying to quickly lose unwanted weight. However, bootcamps can cause a lot of trouble if they involve too much starvation in combination with strenuous exercise. When you don't eat enough, your body tries to do less because it is starving. When you combine this with asking it to do a lot more work and repair due to demanding exercise, it results in what the medical world calls relative energy deficiency syndrome or "REDS." Imagine it is like your whole-body capacity gauge moving into the RED zone. You are asking your body to do more but giving it less to do it with!

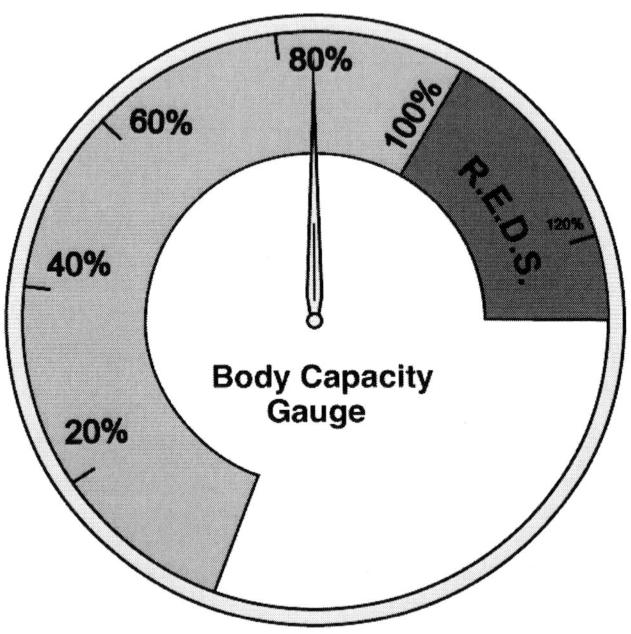

REDS was first described in young, mostly female, very fit, athletes who just didn't eat enough. They were underestimating how much food they needed for their high levels of activity and presented with non-healing injuries and/or lack of menstrual periods. In REDS your body stops sending energy to lower priority systems, most noticeably the reproductive, musculoskeletal, and repair systems. In this "over capacity" state there is a high risk of overtraining and pushing injuries into Plan B. If you stay in REDS for a prolonged period, this can cause lifelong damage, just like an astronaut spending a long time in space.

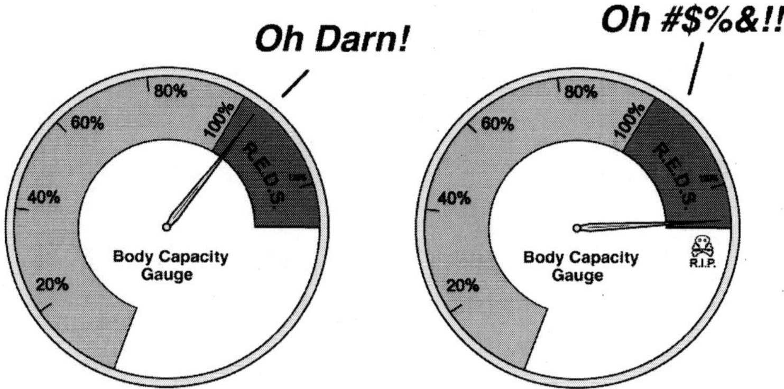

Until I understood what was going on, it was very confusing when slim, middle-aged women came into my clinic with painful osteoarthritic knees but no history of injury or excessive sports in their younger days. The deconditioning event was not immediately obvious to either of us. Further questioning often revealed that several years before, as middle age approached, they had engaged in a prolonged bootcamp style "health kick" to shed "quite a few" pounds. When the possible origin of their problem was discussed, it seemed very unfair to them that all that hard work had caused them trouble in the long run. Surely exercise can never be bad!

Exercise is by far the best medicine for everything, except weight loss. What else can you try? Let's look at diets.

Why Diets Rarely Work in the Long Term

Diet culture is ever-present and can be very damaging. There are hundreds, maybe *thousands*, of diets that promise to be The Diet that will solve weight gain for everyone for the long term.

Unfortunately,

99% of people are back to their pre-diet weight, or even higher, after five years.

I won't go into this topic too deeply, other than to explain my opinion on why one diet, or lifestyle, or strategy will not work for everyone, or even for most people.

By now in this book, you know that we all share commonalities in how our bodies function. You also know that you are unique. The person you are today can never be replicated. You got to where you are today by using your inherited genetic code to customize everything about yourself to the circumstances you grew up in. You continue to fine-tune these adaptations in adult life. If you could magically change your childhood, you would be a similar but different person.

Your body's "food adaptations" are a catalogue of *what you ate in the past*. The habit flywheel applies here too! The foods you have adapted to eat are unique to you, and your preferences stem from childhood. How often you eat certain foods and the length of time you have been eating these foods for may have produced very heavy and fast-spinning flywheels. This means that if you want to change your eating habits, say swap out mac and cheese for salad, or sugary drinks for water (basically slowing down and stopping that flywheel so you can change it), you can experience powerful pushback.

Diets are usually created when someone, somewhere, figured out a way to lose weight and maybe even turned it into a way of life. Often it was not even their own doing. Many diets start with a celebrity who has had their habits managed by a coach or a personal trainer. When this happens, the creator or promoter of the diet gathers "before-and-after" photos, writes a book with detailed instructions, becomes a public speaker, and offers expensive programs that follow what worked for them. They rarely wait to publish, which means the five-year results are not in when they share their "dramatic" transformation.

This is a huge pet peeve of mine. I get tired of young twenty- or thirty-somethings boasting about how they can eat what they want, party all night, and still look fantastic. Or how they have found the magic solution for everybody. Anyone who says, "just do what I do, and you can be like me," doesn't understand that we are all unique. One size does not fit all.

When I hear people boasting or making impossible promises, I think: *Big ****ing deal! When I was younger, I could do that too! I am not twenty anymore so **** off! Stop hurting me and making me feel so $#*%!* (I realize that you could be nodding in agreement right now, or you could be thinking how jealous, bitter, and old I am. Maybe I'm all three).

There is no mystery to how diets work. Essentially, they have the same strategy: Eat less food than your body needs and make it dip into its energy stores. There are literally thousands of ways to do this. They are often dressed up in pseudoscience, wacky ingredients, and promises of magical transformations.

The first problem with diets is that your *body hates starvation*. It is not an efficient state to be in. Most diets go beyond the initial "fasting state," which is more like a rest for your digestive system, and push your body into full-blown rescue mode, which is starvation. From a "whole-body capacity" perspective you can see why starvation may not be good for you. Just as being unfit limits available oxygen, starvation limits available fuel and resources. You are forced to burn your precious, hard-earned fat stores. Who likes having to dip into their rainy day fund?

The other problem is that people who create diets likely have different habits, beliefs, activities, traumas, lifestyles, and cultures than you. A particular diet may work for that person, and all diets *will* work for you in the *short term*, but the habit flywheel is against you. As soon as you fall off the wagon and fail, which is almost inevitable, you will likely revert back to what you did before. Or worse, once you fail it may be easier to justify all those "naughty" things your adapted body has been missing out on and craving. Your well-established food habit flywheels are slow to run down.

There is also so much shame that comes with failing a diet plan. You are left blaming yourself, thinking that if you had just tried harder and completed the program, it would have worked. The failure is seen as yours and not the shortcomings of the revolutionary new diet plan. If you have tried a diet and it didn't work, or you couldn't maintain it, *this is not your fault*. You are simply a different person to the person who made it, and it did not work for you. Later in the book I will help you figure out what will work for you.

How Cravings Play a Role in Weight Gain

This book is about principles. When you understand the underlying principle of efficiency and learn how to listen to what your body is telling you, things start to make more sense. When it comes to your digestive system, your body sends you pain after eating damaging food or just too much food. Your emotions also give you information about what your digestive system hormones are up to. They tell you when you are hungry or full. They even give you cravings that prompt you to eat food that contain resources you need. This is why you feel thirsty and why food tastes so good when you are hungry. Pregnant women are famous for having weird cravings to supply the baby with what it needs. Our hormones can lead us to crave food for other automatic functions if we are growing, stressed, injured, etc.

Let's be honest, eating food makes us feel good. The hormones that control our food consumption become closely blended with other hormones, to give us so many customized emotions that centre around food. We use food not just for fuel and resources, but to celebrate and self soothe; for pleasure, relaxation, and tradition; as a treat; and for so many other reasons.

When you eat something regularly, your body adapts to digesting, processing, and using that food. This builds a habit flywheel for the content of this food. Once the flywheel is spinning your body comes to expect these resources. If it doesn't get them, you experience a craving for that food. Remember this craving can be for food that may be "good" or "bad" for you.

Running on "Rocket Fuel"

Refined sugar is an example of a substance that many of us crave. It has multiple effects on the body, and these effects increase with the volume you consume. Refined sugar is a highly processed carbohydrate that has become the centre of our western food culture. I'm not a conspiracy theorist, but this is one of those times when I believe that society has acted badly. The food and drug industries have often made profit a higher priority than the public's wellbeing. These industries are efficient too. Our dependence on sugar in our culture has been actively developed.

Refined sugar is very easy for the human body to process because it is quickly absorbed into the blood and transported through the body without requiring the whole expensive digestion process. From an efficiency perspective, refined sugar is fantastic, and our bodies let us know. When you eat sugar, you feel the effects almost instantly. You could even say that sugar has its own emotion. Some people call it a "sugar buzz" or a "sugar high."

Of course, there is a problem with this energy source.

Refined sugar is not something that exists in nature. It is a manufactured substance, just like a drug.

This means our bodies are not programmed to handle refined sugar. It is very easy to eat more sugar than our bodies can use, which leads our bodies to store it away in the bank account for a rainy day that will likely never come.

When you consume sugar, your body tries to guess how much sugary food will be coming though the digestive system. Natural sugars tend to need a more involved digestive process as they need to be broken up before they can be absorbed. Refined sugar is ready for direct absorption.

Your body does not seem to know to make the distinction between refined sugar and natural sugars. It seems to always expect the harder-to-digest natural sugars. As refined sugar gets absorbed quickly without digestion it causes a big sugar spike in the blood. Your body mis-interprets this. A sugar spike should mean that there is a large load of natural sugar to process.

Too much sugar in the blood can cause damage. Diabetes shows us that high blood sugars cause havoc in the long term. Because of this, your body turns its sugar storage machinery up to the max. It is efficiently trying to limit these potentially damaging sugar levels by quickly packing it all away in storage. It starts to store sugar immediately but the machinery takes some time to fully ramp up. By the time it is running fast enough to process the large amount of natural sugar it's expecting, the actual smaller amount of refined sugar has already been stored. As no more sugar is being digested and with the storage machinery now running on max, your body starts to store sugar essential for its normal energy needs. This causes the blood sugar level to go lower than required for normal body function.

Low blood sugar is even worse, as you can go unconscious if you don't fuel your heart and brain! As blood sugar levels drop, the storage machinery is shut down, but it is too late. Your blood sugars are now below normal operating levels and your body reports that you urgently need more sugar!

After eating a candy bar, you feel a sugar buzz, because your blood sugar has rapidly risen. With lots of energy available you feel ready to do anything. Within minutes, however, the sugar buzz is usually followed by a "sugar crash" as your body over-does the sugar storage. Your blood sugar suddenly plummets, leaving you feeling sluggish. Even though you have taken on enough energy, all this energy is stored away and is no longer available; you now crave another candy bar! This can be a bumpy existence of highs and lows. Ask anyone who drinks a lot of sugary pop how it feels when they run out or try to stop drinking pop.

Obviously the longer this goes on, and the more refined sugar you consume, the *more adapted* to using refined sugar your body becomes.

Most of us are highly adapted to high sugar diets.

Refined sugar is one the cheapest and most available food ingredients in our culture. It's hidden in the most unlikely food products, adding flavour for cheap. Why is it so bad to run on refined sugar? On top of the bumpy existence of emotional highs and lows until you get your next sugar hit, high blood sugar can be really hard on your body.

Running your body on refined sugar is a bit like running your car on rocket fuel.

If you could run your car on rocket fuel, it would feel great to have all that power. However, running your car hard all the time would probably cause it to wear out prematurely or even tear itself apart. You would also need to refuel it regularly because the fuel would be quickly used up.

In a similar way, adapting and running your sugar digestive machinery to the max can literally wear it out prematurely. Too much of anything can be bad and high blood sugar levels are damaging to all your body's machinery. If you want to understand the long-term effects of too much sugar, look at diabetes. A diabetic's continually damaging high blood sugar levels can be a real capacity hog and may cause body systems to fail much sooner.

Our bodies are more like *multifuel-burning cars*. They run on carbohydrates, fats, and proteins. Most whole foods are combinations all of these. Your body is very adaptable and can even run on other fuels, including alcohol! If you train your body to run primarily on refined sugar, switching to other fuels can be a tough transition. If there is always sugar in the system, it is not efficient to keep the machinery to run your body on fat. This is a real shame, as your body has worked so hard to build up and maintain its emergency store of fat.

Let Them Eat Cake

Everybody loves cake, ice cream, doughnuts, and literally deep-fried anything. Carbohydrate soaked in fat is delicious. This processed food combination cannot be found in nature, but we love it! I have watched hours of TV programs devoted to this delicious food from all around the world. I am literally salivating as I write this. Our bodies seem to have less control when it comes to eating this package of carbohydrate and fat yumminess. Mmmm, pizza ... where's that menu?

This combination delivers "instant fat storage." It packages fat in a coating of instant energy: sugar. This gives your body its favourite long-term investment: fat, wrapped in the energy it needs to run the machinery to store it. No wonder it tastes so awesome and we instantly bond with it! It is like an e-transfer or a direct debit. It goes straight into your bank account with minimum effort. Your body seems to have no "that's enough" mechanism for this kind of transaction. "How could you eat that whole box of doughnuts?!" This can be a very dangerous food group for some of us, needing deliberate self-control. As we all know, junk food is not the best food to run your machine on. Darn it.

Most of us aren't hummingbirds...

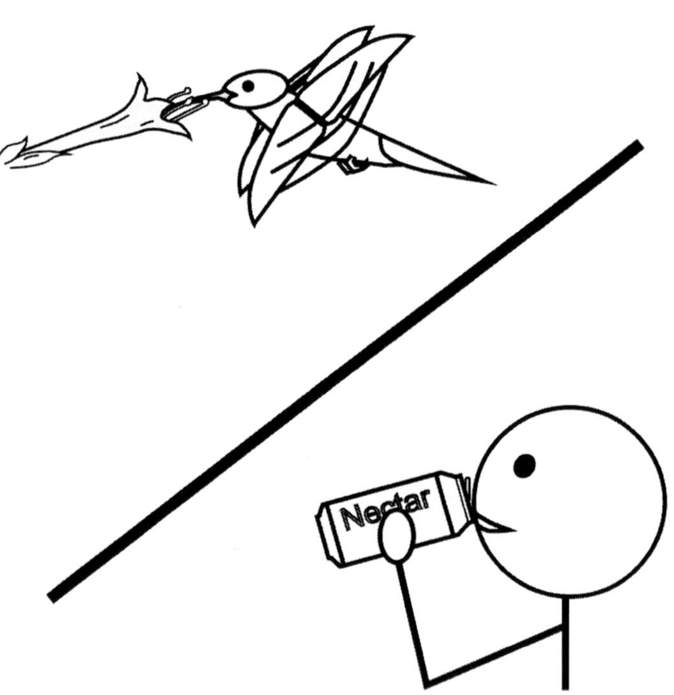

High sugar diets are not for everyone!

Your Weight Can Sneak Up on You

The reasons we gain unwanted weight are many because our relationship with food is learned, complex, and personal. We all overindulge at times. Our body's efficiency ensures that it holds onto as many resources as it can. Even if you only overeat at celebrations four times per year and gain a single pound at each, if you never lose it, you will be 4 pounds heavier by the end of the year. You can say you eat healthily 99 per cent of the time, but you will still be 4 pounds up. This *episodic weight gain* over ten years will result in you being 40 pounds heavier and questioning where the extra weight came from.

Just like breaking a bone or catching a bug, you can overload your digestive system. The greater the overload, the greater the consequences; we will think about these in Chapter 23. You can overload the digestive system to a point where you can't "fix it" on your own. Your body's digestive and storage systems are complex pieces of machinery. They can go wrong like any other part of your body. If caught early enough, there is a way back, but if there is too much damage or overload, you may need rescuing with medications or even surgery.

If you have pushed your sugar machinery to the limit, medications can help you eke a bit more time out of it by pushing it even harder. If you have passed a certain threshold of fat stores there may be no way back without a lot of help. Bariatric surgery can be used in such circumstances, to effectively "ruin your stomach" by stapling (or banding) it smaller or bypassing it all together. Neither medications or surgery are without consequences but should be considered as rescues when you are in a "no win" situation.

Well, What the &$%@ Can I Do to Lose Unwanted Weight?

This chapter may appear quite depressing and full of bad news. I often tell my patients that trying to lose weight in our carbohydrate-worshipping culture is a bit like trying to rehabilitate an alcoholic living in a liquor store. It is not impossible, but it is very hard!

In the next chapter we are going to use your body's principles to discuss how you can work with your body if you want to lose some unwanted weight. It has worked for me for over five years now. You may see it as a passing fad but let's look at why intermittent fasting may be the answer.

Chapter 22

INTERMITTENT FASTING

We all fast. If you eat breakfast ("break-fast") you have fasted overnight. However, most people think of a fast as skipping a meal or two. As we've learned, most diets work against you by putting your body into a prolonged energy deficit. Your body down-regulates its energy needs in a predictable way to try to conserve its valuable energy reserves. We will now discuss how intermittent fasting uses your body's principle of efficiency, to work with you, to achieve sustainable, weight loss. It may even help you to be healthier too.

What's So Great about Fasting?

If starvation is bad, how can fasting (short-term starvation) be good? Fasting can be considered as the first stage of starvation, and it generally means starving your body for a day or two at most. When you do this your body starts to conserve energy, and this can be good for you.

Here is a story to illustrate intermittent fasting. Imagine your work hours have been reduced for a couple of weeks, and your income drops as a result. You know this is a short-term problem.

The first thing you will do is look for ways to save some cash. If you have clothes that you are wearing out, you may repair them instead of replacing them with new ones. You might eat what you already have in your cupboards rather than buying more food.

Your body does the same thing. When in *fasting mode*, it has less ready energy and has to make savings. This is like your phone going into *low power* mode when the battery is running down. You will likely feel a little tired and hungry as you run out of the ready carbohydrates that are usually around. You may be so hangry that nobody wants you around! If you don't usually fast, your body is not adapted to burning fat, so it can't touch your stored fat reserves yet. It takes a couple of weeks to build the machinery to burn fat and utilize the fat reserves.

As your body runs out of available energy, it needs to find some immediate savings. Part of your body's short-term energy saving plan is to repair cells instead of making new cells. *So what?* I hear you ask. *Aren't new cells better than repaired cells?*

Your "physiological age" is a function of how many times your cells have replicated themselves.

We are biological machines with a limited capacity. There is a limit to how many times your body can replicate its cells. You have *thirty trillion cells* in your body and generally each cell can only r*eplicate itself about forty times before it "self-destructs."* This programmed cell death is called "apoptosis." It is a protection against your cells becoming cancer cells. When a cell copies itself, it makes mistakes. The more times it does this, the more mistakes make it through to the new cells. This isn't a big deal unless you do it a lot. After forty replications it appears that the risk goes up, so your cell does the honourable thing.

Your cancer risk is also a function of this process. This means that repairing cells instead of making new cells can be a good idea. In the short term, it is not as ideal as making a new cell but in the long term it can make your body last longer and lower your cancer risk!

How Can Intermittent Fasting Lead to Weight Loss?

Just as to save money you must spend less than you earn, to lose extra weight you must take in less energy than you burn. While you do this, you want to avoid the full-blown starvation that most diet plans put you in, which limits how much your body can do. In the long term, if you continue to starve your body, it adapts by becoming even more efficient. If your body starts trying to do things as cheaply as possible, there can be problems. Just like in the musculoskeletal system, Plan B is initiated when your body realizes it is experiencing a failed healing situation.

Our bodies don't actually need food every day, just like a pack of wolves in the wild will not get a kill every day. Having food available whenever we want is a modern phenomenon. Up until recently, there were no supermarkets and your body's fat stores were very important. For most of human history, we ate when we could, built up our fat storage, and then our bodies burned through this storage until we could find more food. Essentially, to burn fat, you need the machinery to burn fat. Because we never *need* to burn fat in the modern age, we downgrade and may even lose that machinery for efficiency reasons.

Short-term starvation used to be a part of normal life, and your body works best if you run it this way. Fasting is a way to replicate this without causing harm. If you fast regularly, you can tip your body's overall energy balance into deficit over a period of time. Consider the effect of fasting for two days a week on your week's total energy input. Your weekly "bank balance" will now be in deficit as you have dipped into some of your fat reserves.

Why Fasting May Be an Easier Change for You

If you're wondering *how* to fast, I have good news! Remember, you already do a short fast overnight between your last meal of the day and your first one the following morning. This means it's relatively easy to train your body to fast for longer periods. If you do this regularly, your body gets better at it. When you consistently run out of carbohydrates your body retools its fat burning "ketones" metabolism to burn its fat stores.

This is what you can try. Eat supper and then the next morning see how long you can go before you feel wobbly and need to eat. This may be just after breakfast or may be a bit longer. Once you feel this way, eat normally for the rest of the day. Try this once or twice a week, each time seeing if you can go a little longer. Aim to slowly lengthen your fast over the coming weeks and months. Over time, you will find that, even though you may feel a little hungry, you can go longer and longer. Your body will start to invest in its fat-burning metabolism.

This is all you have to do. You do not need to fast for more than a day at a time, or your body will progress into the next stage of its starvation program. This involves turning down systems (including healing) even more. This is less desirable.

It seems that if you fast for a short period on a regular basis your body starts to trust that food is coming again soon. It's like the farmer who tells his accountant not to panic when his bank account is getting low in the summer, because the farm pay cheque comes once a year after the harvest is in. The payoff is that your body learns to burn fat and during the fasting period repairs cells instead of making new ones.

A rule of thumb is that a sixteen-hour fast is enough to get your body to repair cells. If you are trying to shed some unwanted fat, a twenty-four-hour fast is enough to get it to dip into its fat reserves. By doing this a couple of times a week, you will naturally decrease 25–30 per cent of your weekly calorie intake, which should lead to some weight loss. The only requirement is that you continue to eat your usual amount on your non-fasting days. Most people naturally do this anyway.

While fasting can be a great thing to do, there are times when any sort of "diet" is not a good idea. If you are trying to heal an injury, focusing on giving your body enough of the right kind of food is more important. Make sure you are taking in enough energy and resources to heal. I often tell people, that it is ok to put on a pound or too while they are trying to heal an injury. Not an excuse to eat junk though. Darn it.

When deciding where to start and how this can work for you, consider what you are trying to achieve. Personally, I do a sixteen-hour "repair" fast most days from 8 pm to 12 pm the next day. That is supper to lunch. I'm still figuring out how often I need to do this to maintain my fat-burning skills. When I party and pile on a few pounds I do a couple of twenty-four-hour "fat burn" fasts a week, until I get back to where I want to be.

I have not had to change what food I eat at all, and so this strategy has been easy and effective for me.

If This Is Not for You

If intermittent fasting does not sound fun, or if you have tried it in the past, didn't enjoy the experience one bit, and didn't see the results you wanted ... don't worry! Try to find something else that works for you. You could seek professional advice. If you prefer to work it out for yourself, there are thousands of ways to starve yourself and thousands of books documenting the journey.

Healthy Eating

A final note on a common mistake that people make. Eating healthy food is not the same as trying to shed unwanted weight. The idea that eating a bit of lettuce will fix everything is a mistake I have made too. Remember that from an efficiency perspective

Healthy food gives you the energy and raw materials you need, whilst doing the minimal amount of damage.

Generally, the less processed food is, the less garbage comes with it. Imagine what has happened to your food on its journey to you. The less stuff it has had added to it and the less it has been messed with, the less likely it is to hurt you and the more likely it is to be better for you. Even if you eat less of the garbage and more of the healthy stuff, you will still not lose weight until you put your body into starvation mode.

You can lose weight eating junk food. This is still not the best idea though. Darn it.

I will get into habit change and my own weight-loss journey in Part 5. This is a story of fumbling around incompetently until someone helped me! Before we reach the more practical part of this book I want to talk about what happens when you exceed your whole body's capacity. At some point in all our lives, our bodies just have too much to do.

Chapter 23

EXCEEDING YOUR BODY'S CAPACITY

"That's all I can stands, I can't stands no more!"

Popeye sums it up. There's only so much abuse you can take. There is an upper limit to everything we do. We have learnt that this is true for your body as a whole. So, when you do go over capacity and your body can't fix everything anymore, what does it do?

When You Overload Multiple Systems, Which Is Repaired First?

As you learned with sensation gating, prioritizing is very important to your body. This mechanism goes beyond sensations and emotions, impacting how the systems in your body function.

Your body has limited resources, and it uses them efficiently to keep you functioning to the best of your ability.

When you are young, healthy, and uninjured, you rarely give your body more to do than it can do. You can party all night and still get up for work the next day. However, when you have an injury, and as you get older, resources that are used for your normal daily operation tasks are reallocated for repair. When multiple systems are overloaded at the same time, things start to get complicated. What happens when you exceed your body's capacity to do everything? Just like anyone with too much on their "to-do" list, your body must prioritize.

How do we know which body systems are the most important? Just like anything in life, if you want to find out how important something is, consider what happens if you *don't* do it. Let's play a game and consider the consequences of "turning off" different bits of your body.

First let's turn off your heart, lungs, or brain. How long would you live? Only a few minutes before you are deceased, "brown bread dead," have "kicked the bucket," or "shuffled off this mortal coil." You can deduce that these are essential systems.

Next, consider turning off your liver, spleen, kidney, or guts. How long would you live? Generally, a few days to a few weeks. These are less important systems, but still important for ongoing survival. Let's say they are medium priority systems.

What about your musculoskeletal system or your reproductive system? If you lose an arm, a leg, or your ovaries or testicles, you may not feel like carrying on, but you can still live a normal length life. These are therefore low-priority, or non-essential, systems.

An Example from Intensive Care

Think about what happens if you get really sick and end up in the intensive care unit in the hospital. Because you are fighting for your life your body has too much to do. Your body prioritises sending energy to your heart, lungs, and brain. As it diverts energy to your high priority systems, the lower priority ones lose out. Blood flow decreases to your arms and legs, limiting their function. Next your guts, liver, and kidneys get less energy and may start to shut down. If you are incredibly sick, even your brain goes into "low power mode" and you fall unconscious, which is involuntary sleep. If you are sick for long enough, your body sends so little energy to low priority "distant parts," like your fingers and toes, that they die and fall off! When the battle is lost, your heart, lungs, and brain finally shut down. The end. Essentially, your body stops supporting systems in a predictable way from the least to the most important.

Normal life account

ACCOUNTS

SPENDING	$
Brain	-500
Digest food	-230
Go for run	-600
BUDGET	10,000
TOTAL	8,770

Catastrophic life account

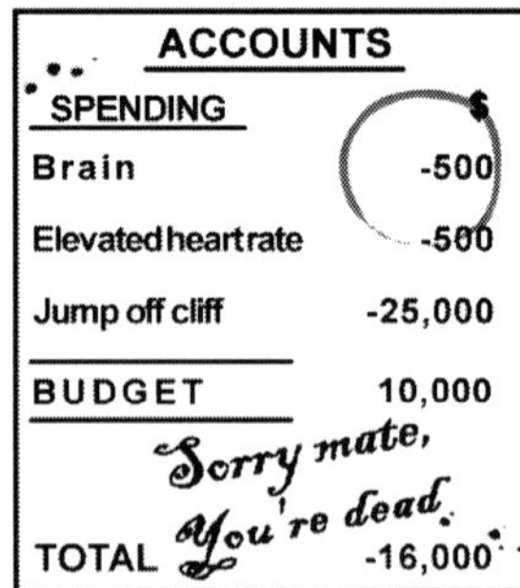

ACCOUNTS

SPENDING	$
Brain	-500
Elevated heart rate	-500
Jump off cliff	-25,000
BUDGET	10,000
TOTAL	-16,000

Why Are Plumbers So Hard to Find?

Imagine that you have a crew of white cell workers that do all the repairing in your body. You can think of them as tiny robots. Every day they are sent around your body to do maintenance and repairs based on a list of jobs. This to-do list is always prioritized depending on what is the most important to fix. This means that if all is going well, they have a simpler day and can put their resources into repairing minor things like a cut finger or a bruised shin. Their day gets busier when unexpected things happen.

Let's compare them to a crew of plumbers with a list of tasks to do each day. Since there are only so many plumbers, they can only do so much work. Today, one homeowner wants new central heating installed, so they all set off to install the new central heating.

As they start the job, an emergency call comes in. A pipe has burst in another house, and it needs urgent repair. The boss leaves a couple of workers to install the central heating and takes most of the crew to fix the burst pipe. While they are fixing the pipe, another call comes in. A hot water tank has burst in another house. The boss now calls the crew that was installing the central heating to go to this new emergency. By the end of the day, the two emergencies are under control, but the central heating is not installed. Perhaps they will get that job done tomorrow. However, the next day begins with another emergency call for a burst pipe ... Some days you just can't get a plumber.

Your body works in the same way.

Your body prioritizes the most important repair in the most important systems first.

If you have a lot of things going on at the same time, some systems will never get the resources they need to repair quickly. The lower priority systems lose out.

Your body is limited in its resources for repair, and overload gets harder to stay on top of with age. When you are young you can do a lot. You can run your body hard and have capacity to spare. As you get older that capacity slowly declines. There comes a day when your body just can't do everything.

The Effects of Smoking

With all of this in consideration, let's look at the effects of cigarette smoking. Did you know that smokers do not heal as quickly as non-smokers? If they get a flu or injure themselves, they repair slower than a non-smoker with the same overload. By now, you may understand why.

Cigarette smoke contains carbon monoxide. This sticks to your body's hemoglobin, which is used to transport oxygen in the blood. A smoker's body is not able to carry as much oxygen to the tissues to burn fuel. It is like having a dirty air filter on your car engine. The body's overall capacity to do work is reduced. Importantly, smoking damages *essential* systems (the lungs and heart), which are prioritized over other injuries.

This means that if you are a smoker and you're trying to get stronger at the gym, you will not repair and upgrade your muscles as quickly as a non-smoker. It also means that if you drop a weight on your foot and have to wear a cast, your injury will not repair as quickly or fully as a non-smoker's injury would. Sometimes a break or fracture becomes a "fracture non-union" and it doesn't heal at all!

If you are a smoker and you catch a bad flu while laid up on the couch with your broken foot, your sickness will linger for longer and your bone will be a big deal to heal! You risk getting pneumonia or having a broken bone that does not heal at all. Your precious, limited resources are being diverted to repair the continual damage in your higher priority lungs.

Smoking is a very large investment of your body's resources. It's like that mortgage on the house you can't really afford. You'd better really love that house! You may find that although you enjoy owning it, you may not be able to afford to maintain it or do other things you want to. In Part 5, I will share a story about a smoker who wants to stop smoking. Like any habit with a powerful flywheel, this is a tough one to change, but it is within your power to do so.

The Whole-Body Effects of Too Much ________

Fill in the blank. Too much of a good thing can be bad. Just as smoking can be taxing on your resources, so can carrying too much fat. Imagine you must pay for storing money in a bank account. Most of us object to the bank charging us for looking after our money, but there is a cost involved. Maintaining your fat reserves is expensive too. Unlike a bank account, not only do you have to keep your fat reserves alive and healthy, but you also have to carry them around with you.

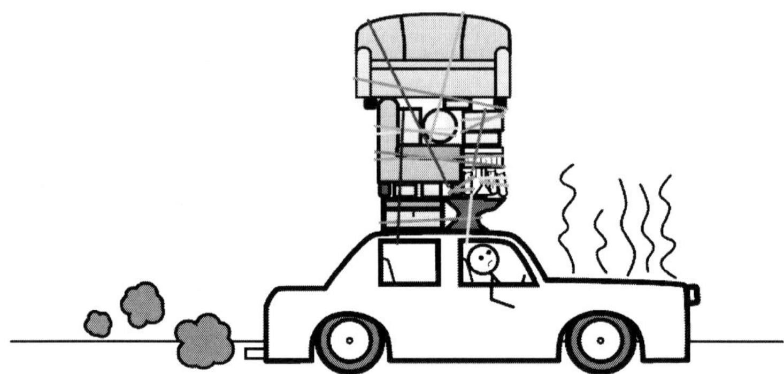

Perhaps I'm carrying too much weight...

Imagine carrying 100 litres of fuel in containers in the trunk of your car just in case you run out. Your car would have to work harder, and it would wear out quicker. In a similar way, the extra work required to carry and maintain stored fat is taken away from your body's daily operating capacity. If you have a lot of fat stored and you are working within capacity, all is well. If one day you go over capacity, by getting sick or injured, things can go wrong quickly.

Going over capacity can be like falling off a cliff.

You can be a relatively "healthy" smoker, alcoholic, drug addict, or extreme skier (fill in your "bad" behaviour of choice) by operating *within* your body's capacity. As long as you are not overloading your body too much and sending your "plumbers" into a flurry all day long, things go reasonably well.

This means not getting sick, not getting too stressed out, and not working your body too hard.

However, when you live on the edge, it only takes one problem to tip you over capacity. There are many things that put us at risk of this. A smoker who is functioning just fine can get COVID, and everything goes downhill. An alcoholic can start smoking too, and this habit is enough for them to remain over capacity for the foreseeable future. Risk adds up. An extreme skier takes a lot of risks (their good luck capacity) and one day that close call becomes a bad fall. As we get older, at some point we all go over capacity. How likely you are to fall depends on how close to the edge of the cliff you are.

The Over-Capacity "Warning Light"

Most of my work is with pain in the musculoskeletal system, which is a lower-priority system. When your body goes over capacity, one of the first things it stops fixing is the musculoskeletal system. This means that ongoing pain in my line of work is a common problem! When I encounter musculoskeletal injuries that are not healing, I look for reasons why this person is over capacity.

Often the reason is, unfortunately, ageing, which is inevitable. However, in a younger person there is another reason. Maybe they are overweight, a smoker, or struggling with a deconditioning event, such as an injury. More essential systems such as the guts and lungs will always be repaired before their musculoskeletal injury. It is more helpful to first address the problems in the "higher priority systems" and often the musculoskeletal injury will then heal without much further intervention.

This all has implications if you are trying to change something! Some things are harder to change than others. Often a good place to start is to consider what you can change now to free up some of those resources in your body, those workers that help repair and create change. For example, you could stop smoking. You could increase your fitness so your body can do more of everything. If you are an athlete, make sure you are eating enough food to fuel your training. Another thing you can do is get better sleep.

The Magic of Sleep

Have you ever asked yourself why you need to sleep? It can feel like such a waste of time. Being awake is much more exciting! The truth is that being awake is expensive for your body. Your brain alone uses 20 per cent of your available fuel when you are awake. Moving around burns fuel. Digesting food burns fuel. Everything you do needs fuel.

Your body fixes some of the things on its to-do list during the day, but most of it gets fixed while you sleep. The overload that happens during the day mostly gets repaired and potentially upgraded at night. Even your brain learning operates on this principle. If you are studying for a test and do not sleep, you do not learn. Your brain changes by making new connections between nerves, which is a form of repair! This is why the advice to "sleep on it" when you need to solve a problem actually works.

Sleep is your body's maintenance time.

When you are unconscious, you are no longer consciously working your systems. During this important break, your body can redirect its resources from its expensive essential systems to give less important parts the chance to fix. Sleep is not an energy-saving time, as some people think, but a time to redirect resources for repairing and upgrading.

Remember the intensive care unit in the hospital. When you are badly injured or sick, the most important tool doctors have is to turn off your conscious brain and support your body's systems with life-support machines and drugs. When the number of things you need to fix puts your body catastrophically over capacity, it is at risk of failing completely. Artificially giving you extra capacity allows you to survive and fix things you could not fix on your own. A less dramatic ICU is your bed! There is a strong argument for saying that *sleep is the best medicine!* The restoration of sleep can feel like magic. Enough good quality sleep plays a very important role in preventing you from going over capacity.

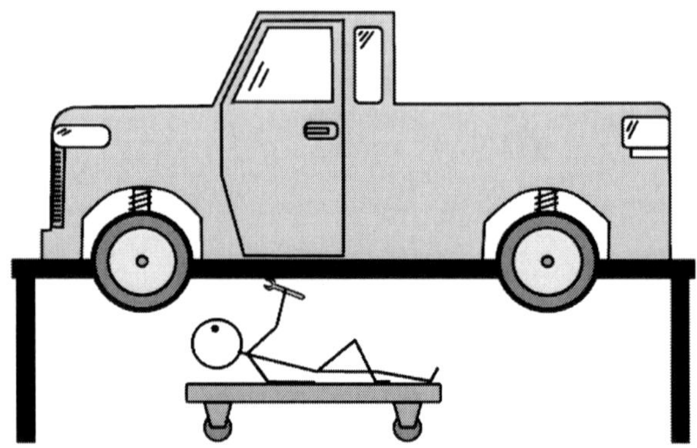

Repair and Upgrade

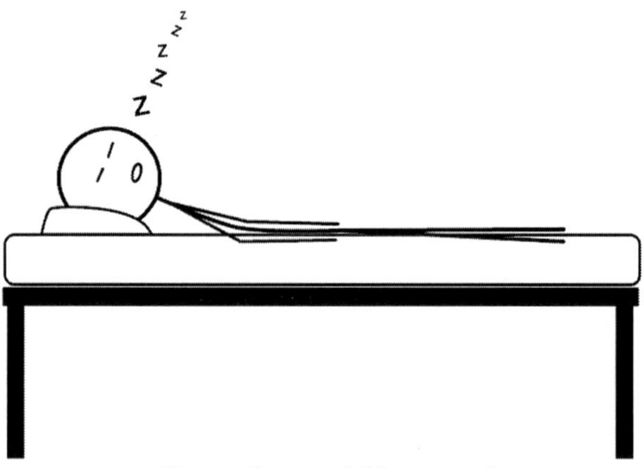

Repair and Upgrade

Sleeping is something you can learn to get better at too! You may need to get some help to improve your "sleep hygiene." Don't be afraid to educate yourself or even better get advice from a sleep expert. Good sleep can feel like heaven. Poor sleep can feel like hell.

Chapter 24

YOUR LIFETIME CAPACITY

We are biological machines that wear out predictably. You adapt yourself through childhood by what you do with your inherited genetic information. Your body is trying to guess what you are going to do for the rest of your life. When you stop growing and become an adult your body has customized you for the future, and you are like a brand-new car driving off the showroom forecourt. From that moment on, you start to wear out.

You customize your machine as a child.
As an adult you can renovate but you can't rejuvenate.

Imagine two identical, brand-new cars. They each have a potential capacity. What happens to them once they are driven off the lot determines how they will wear out. If one is turned into a rally car and the other one is left stock and potters around town, they will look very different twenty years later. The specialized rally car will have different problems from the family wagon, but eventually both will suffer wear and tear. The same is true for our bodies. No matter how much we try to maintain our youth, turn back time, or ignore the effects of age, the slow wearing down of our bodies is a core principle of how our body works.

How a car wears out is predictable. Whether it reaches its "potential capacity" is based on "what it gets up to" and how well it is maintained. The same is also true for your body. Remember

You're free to choose whatever you like in life, but you're not free from the consequences of those choices.

It's up to you to choose to work with your body, not against it.

The Importance of Proper Maintenance

Failing to maintain a car with good quality fuel, regular oil changes, tire pressures checks, fluid level checks, washing, and polishing can lead to parts failing prematurely. It is the same for your human machine. Not maintaining your body with proper food and rest can cause premature failure, especially if you are going to run it hard. The most important maintenance you can do for your body is allowing for adequate recovery to complete repairs.

Let's compare two runners. They are both dedicated and always take themselves to the limit. The first runner believes that *pain is weakness* and always pushes through discomfort and challenge. He develops an intense training plan with a set schedule, which he is determined to stick to.

The second runner also sets an ambitious schedule but is flexible. She realizes that *recovery is the key* to progressing. Each day she assesses how recovered she is and adjusts her schedule accordingly. Some days she does more than she planned, and some days she does less than she planned. This second runner even takes days off when she doesn't feel fully recovered.

When both athletes are young, they do well. They both seem to have "capacity to spare." But as they get older, differences start appearing. The first runner starts to go over capacity and is no longer completing repairs. He pushes through but his performance tails off.

The second runner finds she needs more recovery time than she used to but keeps adjusting and remains competitive. She is even keeping up with some of the younger athletes who seem to be training harder than she is.

As we fast forward through their lives, we catch up with the first runner in the doctor's office in his early fifties with worn-out knees, wondering what he did wrong. He was always the fittest, hardest working athlete he knew. He tells his doctor, "I haven't done anything different. I've been running like this my whole life! I was told that exercise is the best medicine! This is really ****ing unfair."

Meanwhile, the second runner continues to run and do other activities into her sixties, seventies, and eighties. She is not as fast as in her glory days and she certainly can't keep up with the youngsters anymore, but she's still doing well, experiences little or no pain, and is fulfilled. She modifies her expectations and activities as she ages.

Any competitive sport has the potential to cause you to "wear out" faster. If you do not put an emphasis on recovery in your training, you will wear out even more quickly. It's also true that you can't be a successful athlete without pain. It's all about learning to read your body's signals to know how far and how hard you can push, when to rest, when your body has recovered, and when it is ready to do it again!

As you accumulate wear and tear over time, your capacity drops. Specialization can be a big factor in this process. In the case of both runners, they chose to specialize their bodies through training to run. A consequence of this is that their knees' capacity is used up more quickly than if they had not specialized in running. Specialisation can lead things to wear out quicker, but the consequences can be magnified if the importance of recovery is missed. No pain, no gain but pushing through the pain too much can get you into trouble.

The good news is that you have some control over these capacities. You can increase your overall capacity using individualised training with a focus on recovery. You can maintain your body and help things last longer. You just have to pay attention to what your body is telling you. You can then make informed decisions about what you want to invest your body in.

Your Lifetime Capacity

Everything you do has a capacity. Not just a capacity to do it today, but to do it over a lifetime. Over the years your adult body experiences a slow decline in capacity in every system. However, you can wear out one system quicker than another.

It is possible to use up your lifetime capacity in a system prematurely with too much specialisation. Drinking alcohol is a good example. If you specialise in drinking booze, you can train your liver to process alcohol to the maximum. As you get better at drinking, you can consume more alcohol than other people, with only the same level of drunkenness. Running your liver this hard will have consequences. Even a young adult who consistently gets very drunk without adequate repair time, will run through their lifetime capacity to process alcohol before they even hit middle age. Some young people who regularly binge-drink end up needing a liver transplant in their twenties. Not ideal.

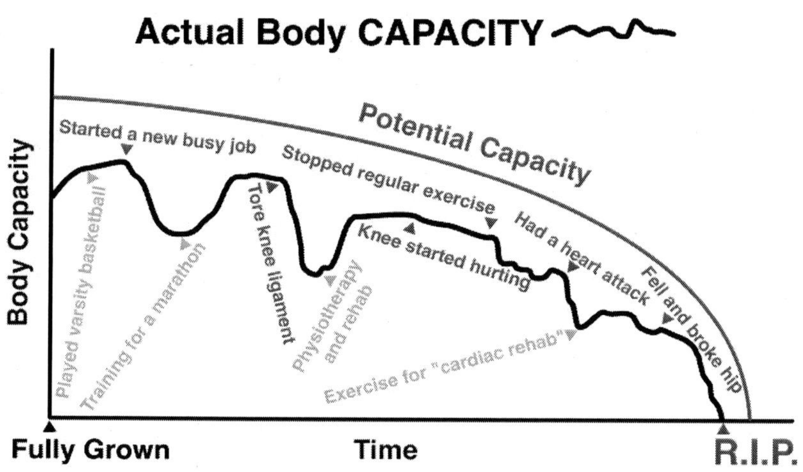

Our lives are one long journey of overload and repair.

If you don't allow for completed repair, you may experience acceleration in the long-term wearing out of your body and face lower-than-expected capacity as you age. Remember, you can choose to live however you want but you are not free from the consequences of those choices! The diversity in people is astonishing. You can meet a sixty-year-old in a long-term care facility unable to walk up the stairs, but you can also meet an eighty-year-old who still hikes in the mountains with their grandkids.

When Age and Ambition Meet

There comes a time in everyone's life when they notice they aren't recovering the way they once did. I call this the time *when age and ambition meet* – when you struggle to meet your ambitions because of your age. We can look to our sporting heroes for some clues as to when this happens.

Most people who dedicate themselves to professional sports train to the max. How many of your sporting heroes are still competing at a high level in their forties? Not many and if they are, they are in the news. Some sports or sporting positions favour the young, like playing a forward position in hockey. Some sports can be played at a high level for longer, like golf. Just look at the average age of retirement in a particular sport to get an idea of how hard it is on your body.

Age and ambition tend to meet at around thirty-five to forty years old. This is the age of people I commonly see in my office with musculoskeletal problems as they are not repairing and have entered Plan B (chronic inflammation mode). They are having a similar capacity problem to an under-eating athlete with REDS (relative energy deficiency syndrome) but age is now the cause. They are experiencing consistent pain as their bodies have too much on their to-do lists. Musculoskeletal complaints are one of the commonest reasons for visiting a health care professional. Now you know why.

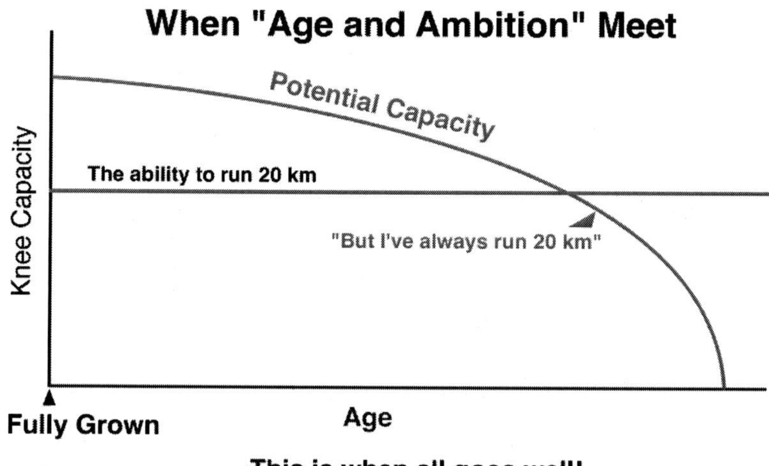

This is when all goes well!

Age and ambition meet when your whole body goes over capacity.

When you hit this crucial midpoint of your life, you have some choices to make. Age and ambition *always* meet eventually. It doesn't matter how well you take care of your body. For some, this turning point is earlier than others. Regardless of when it happens, it does not have to mark the end of doing what you love to do. Just like the second runner in my earlier example, you can make decisions now that will help you make the most of your capacity in the long term.

It is true that specialization will probably lead to paying a price down the road. However, most professional athletes who dedicate themselves to specialization will tell you *it was TOTALLY worth it*. Some will say it wasn't. It is up to you to choose how you use your body.

Your body, your choice!

PART 5

Making a Change

Chapter 25

CHOOSING A CHANGE

Congratulations on making it to the last part of this book. Fanfare! The "putting it all together bit." The "penny drops," "I need to change something" bit. Or possibly you are thinking, "%$&@ #*//, this is a long book!"

Anyhow, let's try to use what we have learned to actually, meaningfully, change something. This is not a "be more like me" plan that you find in so many books. Please *do not* try to be like me. My wife will tell you what a spectacularly bad idea this would be. This is all about you. Please *do* use the principles I have observed to make the most of the "hand you have been dealt."

The good news is that it's never too late to change.

So long as you are breathing, your body is trying to make you better!

However, it's probably not a good idea to leap into changing the first thing that comes into your head. Perhaps you have already tried this in the past! This may go better if you start by taking some time to consider what is the best thing for you to change at this point in your life. This chapter will help lead you through the process of how to choose a good change. You are far more likely to be successful if you make a good choice in the first place. We will look at all the different factors that affect how hard or easy a particular change will be for you, but first I want to get into what habits are and why our body has them.

Why Are Habits Efficient?

We have talked about the habit flywheel that represents activities we do regularly. The longer you have pursued a habit, and the more often you do it, the faster and heavier the habit flywheel spins. In the example of the two brothers who stop running on the same day, I used the habit flywheel to illustrate what happens when you stop doing a *desirable* habit. The brother who runs more often and has been running for longer can get back to his previous capacity quicker than his brother because his flywheel has more momentum and spins down slower.

In this final part of the book, we are going to talk about making a new habit (starting a new flywheel), building on a desirable habit you already have (making a habit flywheel heavier and faster), or winding down an *undesirable* habit like smoking or eating junk ("braking" the flywheel, making it lighter and slower, to "break" the habit).

What are habits for? Because your body is efficient, it is always trying to prepare you for what is going to happen next. Your body cannot see the future, so it uses what has already happened to you to try to predict the future. Has a friend ever said to you, "I knew you were going to do that!"? Just like your friend remembering how you reacted in the past, your body uses what happened to you last time to predict what you are going to do this time. It is much more efficient to build on past experiences than be constantly trying to work out what to do from scratch.

"I like firsts. Good or bad, they're always memorable."
—Ahsoka Tano, The Mandalorian

When something happens to you for the first time, you make a brand-new memory. Your body records or "imprints" this event as foundational memory. A lot of this imprinting happens in childhood. How we imprint a first memory is very important because it can dictate how we use the memory in the future. The actions and consequences of this event are recorded with the memory. If there is a big effect on your life, the memory can be very strong, even if it only happened once. This can be something good, like your first kiss, maybe. It can also be something bad, as previously discussed with PTSD.

PTSD can be the result of a really big, bad event in someone's life. PTSD is an example of imprinting a very powerful memory that causes lasting consequences because it can easily trigger a person to literally relive the bad event in their mind.

Your body efficiently uses imprinted memories to guide future actions.

Actions Are Triggered by Memories

As we go through life our body is constantly creating memories from the situations we find ourselves in. This is a bit like taking photos when you go on a trip. Photos record pictures of events during your trip, but memories also include a snapshot of the "state of your whole body" during that event. Get out some old photos. An old picture will often trigger a memory. That beach photo takes you back to the sea. You feel the wind, taste the ocean, and recall the annoyance you felt at having sand in your underwear. This memory is made up of the recorded event (what happened), the sensations (what you touched, saw, heard, tasted, or smelled), and the emotions you felt during it (happiness, fear, hunger, etc.,). Because there are three parts to every recorded memory, I call it a "memory triad."

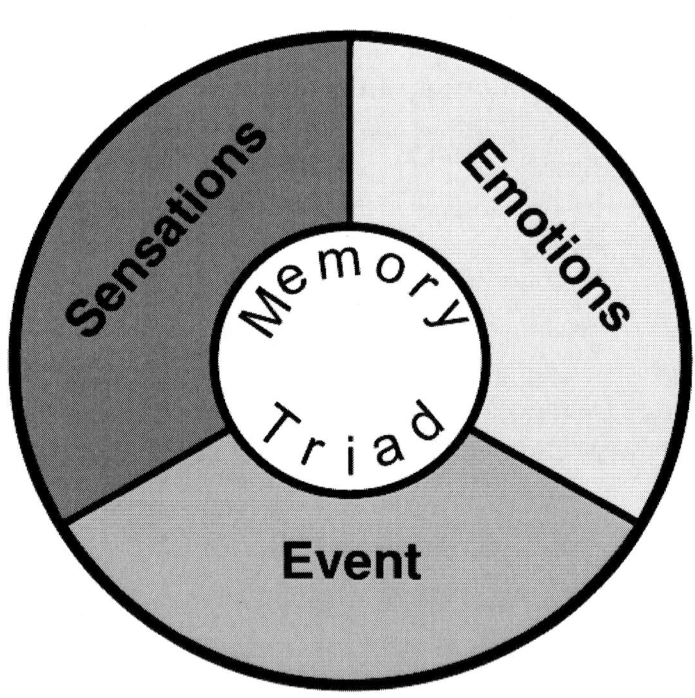

Every situation leads to an action. For example, the beach trip results in you trying to get sand out of your underwear, or a balloon unexpectedly popping at a birthday party makes you jump. This action then has a consequence. We react to that consequence by making a judgement about whether the outcome of this situation is good or bad. Perhaps now you don't like balloons or beaches. We can think of this as our attitude to the memory and its outcome. Our attitude is our interpretation of how we feel about a habit. Some people don't care about the irritating sand because they just love being by the ocean.

A habit is an "action program" that your body runs in response to a memory (any part of the memory triad). For example, when you wake up in the morning you remember that you like coffee. Any part of the *memory triad* can trigger the action – maybe you feel the emotion "groggy" when you wake up, or you experience a familiar sensation like the sound of your alarm, or you perform a routine event such as putting on your slippers and walking into the kitchen. Any of these things can trigger the action program of making yourself a cup of coffee. This program can also be triggered at other times of the day. If you feel groggy in the afternoon or you smell someone else's coffee, this could trigger the action program again. Whether you are aware of how this memory triad is triggered depends on how long you have been doing the triggered habit. Long-standing habits can become automatic.

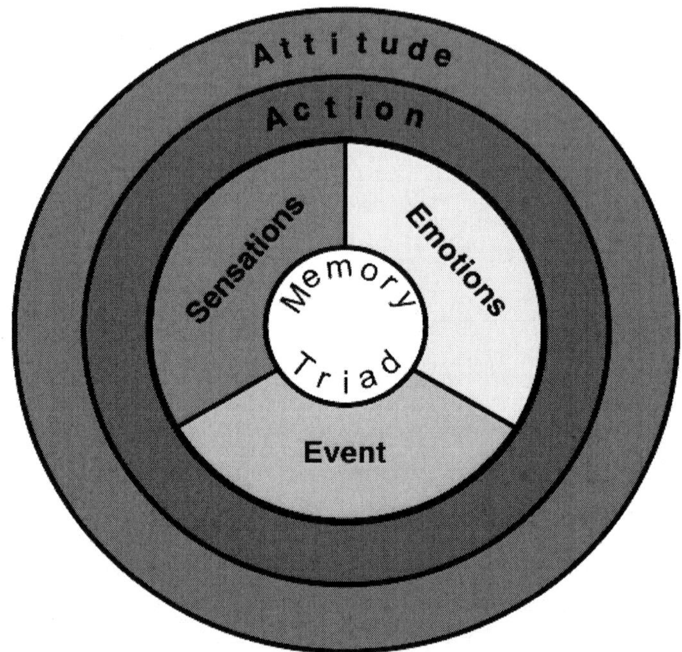

Memory Triad Habit Wheel

Here is the final and most important principle I'm going to share in this book:

Habits allow your body to efficiently get ready to perform an action.

When you experience something new you record it by imprinting a new *memory triad* and associated action. If the impact of this experience is large you can quickly establish a habit. When I first skied I thought it was the most amazing thing ever! The impact of that imprinting was large enough that I have skied at every opportunity since. Habits with a lower impact may take longer to become established. For example, for years I was not a coffee lover and would only drink coffee on some days. When I started shift work, I began to feel the "need" for coffee to wake me up, so I started to drink it more often. Now I "automatically" drink coffee, every single day.

How hard it is to change depends on how well this memory and triggered action (habit) is established.

When you repeat an activity, you are building on an existing memory triad and action. Each time you go through this cycle of recalling a memory and triggering an action, you make the habit stronger. The body starts to invest in this habit flywheel, and it starts to gain habit momentum. Every time you go through this habit cycle your body refines the memory and the action to try to get a better outcome. The more you run this habit, the greater your capacity to do the habit. Remember that you make your muscles bigger by the repetitive habit of regularly training them. You both get better at lifting weights and get bigger muscles. Interestingly, the more you do the activity, the easier it is to trigger as well. The more you train at the gym, the more likely you are to train at the gym.

These memory triads with an action and attitude attached are what makes up the habit flywheels we were thinking about earlier in the book. The weight of the flywheel is your body's ongoing investment in the habit and how fast it spins is determined by how often the habit is triggered and performed. The habit momentum is your capacity to perform the habit at any one time.

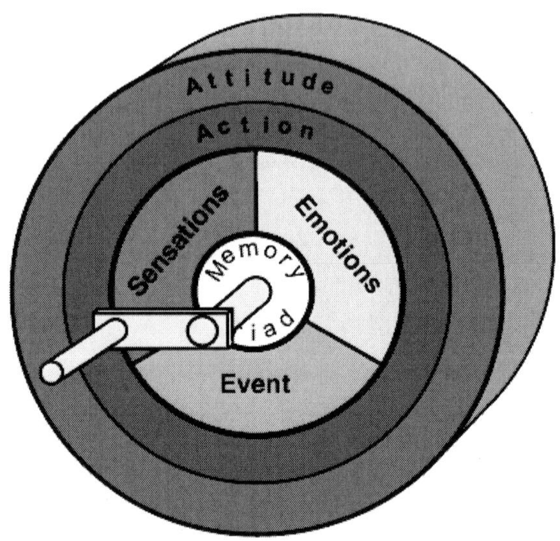

Bringing it all together with the ***Memory Triad Habit Flywheel.***

Now you understand what habits are for and how they are triggered, you are in a better position to consider changing a habit. You may be thinking, *how do I go about this?* It is important to take some time to prepare a successful approach to changing a habit. As Hannibal from the A-Team used to say, after taking the time to create a wildly heroic scheme to save the day with nothing but the junk he found around him:

"I love it when a plan comes together."

Preparing to Make Your Plan

Like Hannibal, doctors make a lot of plans. When I meet a patient in my clinic, my interview involves working out what their problem is and assessing how able they are to make changes to improve the problem. If the complaint is their knee, my consultation starts like this: "I understand that you have a problem with your knee, but you are so much more than just a knee. Let's talk about the rest of you first, then we can talk about the problem with your knee and come up with a plan to help get you better."

What I am doing is taking time to prepare the information I need to work out their "capacity to change," define what their problem is, and finally formulate a realistic plan for them to make changes that will help solve that problem. This differs from the "cookbook," one size fits all, recipe approach to problems that I was originally taught.

If you watch one of those cookery competition shows where they give the contestants three weird ingredients and ask them to make a meal fit for a king, you will notice that the successful chefs take a few minutes to come up with a realistic, customised plan. Those who dive right in or are overly ambitious are rarely successful. In surgical training we are taught a mantra: *Plan well, cut well, get well!* Perhaps we could adapt this and say:

Plan well, change well, stay well!

We will now consider three questions that will help you "plan well" to successfully change a habit and make it stick.

Deciding what to change starts with figuring out what "ingredients you have" and what you can realistically do with them. You probably already have a change in mind, so let's think about that change and how likely you are to be successful at it.

1. How big is the change?

A bigger change will be more difficult and take longer than a smaller change. For example, if you want to eat a healthier diet and you already cook most of your meals and enjoy vegetables, the change will be less drastic. If you avoid cooking like the plague and most of your food comes in pre-prepared packets, or you are on first-name terms with the pizza delivery driver, you will be in for a rougher ride.

How long and how often you have been doing a habit dictates how fast and heavy your habit flywheel has become. If you already have a flywheel spinning, it is easier to get it spinning faster, than to build a brand-new habit flywheel. Generally, the bigger the change you are trying to make the greater the investment required in building up the habit flywheel.

For example, if you want to ride your bike more, the change will be easier if you have been riding your bike twice a week for a year, because you will have more habit momentum, than if you have only been out on your bike twice or not at all. If you want to become a body builder and you already go to the gym four times a week and have a personal trainer, your activity momentum is already very high and the change will be easier for you than if you don't even know where the gym is.

Thinking about what you already do helps you to think about how big the change will be. A drastic change may be going vegan if you are a daily meat eater or learning to play the piano if you have never played an instrument in your life. If the change is quite big, think about ways of making the change in smaller steps. Perhaps cutting out meat for one meal a week or starting to sing along to songs.

Back to that change you were thinking of. Ask yourself, *do I think of myself as the type of person who usually [fill in your desired habit]?* If your answer is no because it is a big departure from what you usually do, it is going to be much harder for you to make this change.

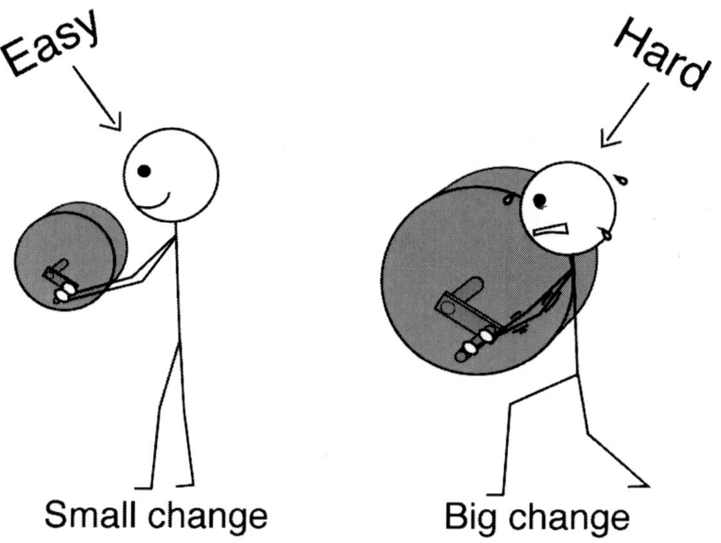

2. How many things are you trying to change?

Trying to change lots of things at once is tempting. Every time a new year rolls around, we tend to make an extensive list of things we want to change. This list of new year's resolutions rarely makes it beyond January. Is the change you are thinking of simple, or are you dreaming of a whole new you?

The problem with making *lots of small changes* is that they all add up to a *big change*. Changes use resources. The more changes you want to make, the more work your body has to do. How many habit flywheels are you trying to change at the same time? Your "change capacity" is going to be divided between all of them. Imagine running between all those different wheels to try to keep them spinning. You can overload your change capacity.

If you are trying to stop one habit and replace it with another, this also counts as changing more than one thing. Imagine trying to stop a very heavy and fast spinning flywheel at the same time as starting another one spinning.

It is very hard to make drastic lifestyle changes stick because you try to change too much, too fast. Beware the "new you by the weekend" type of advice that is so common. Those young influencers who boast about finding the answer are just displaying what you can get away with when you have a youthful body. In the realm of food and exercise, we seem to have culturally adopted an extreme all-or-nothing approach when it comes to change.

Because of this faulty thinking, things like bootcamps and social media challenges have been extremely popular over the years. These schemes are more likely to put you into the REDS zone on your body's capacity gauge. This can increase your risk of injury and the likelihood of pushing you into plan B. Perhaps doing one hundred push ups by the end of the month is not a realistic goal for you!

A common health kick is the combination of a healthier diet, a more active lifestyle, and the loss of some unwanted weight. To be successful it is better to choose just one thing to change at a time. Remember the principle:

Low and slow is the way to go.

Once you have made one small change, you can then move onto the next. Remember lots of completed small, stepwise changes will add up to a big change in the end.

Back to that change you were thinking of. Ask yourself, *how many things am I trying to change?* If your answer is "a lot" then it is going to be much harder for you to make this change.

3. What is your capacity to change?

Your change capacity is the amount your body can change at a given time, and it is affected by the same things that affect your capacity to heal (repair). Imagine your change capacity as how much time and energy you can dedicate to changing your habit flywheels.

Many things can decrease your capacity for change. Your capacity to do everything slowly decreases with age, change is much easier when you are younger! You have probably heard the phrase, "You can't teach an old dog new tricks!" A deconditioning event leading to decreased fitness, or chronic health problems, can decrease change capacity. Additionally, we all have resource hogs to contend with. These are things in your life that require your time and resources to be spent elsewhere, like a stressful or physically demanding job, high-level sports, raising young children, being overweight, regular drinking, or smoking. This leaves less of your energy and resources available to make any change.

Factors that increase your capacity for change might be improving cardiovascular fitness or working on getting better quality of sleep. Do not forget sleep is the most important recovery tool you have! Often, the best way to increase your change capacity is to gain control of and, if possible decrease your resource hogs.

Having a realistic idea of your actual capacity for change helps to give you a better perspective on how tough it may be to make any change. It might be a good idea to focus on increasing your capacity to change first before making other changes. For example, getting fitter means you can then change more of everything. This is the change that makes all other changes easier!

For fun, I've started a table of factors that may increase and decrease your change capacity below. Note that these are the same things that promote your ability to repair.

Look at the table and see how this applies to you. If most of your factors are in the left column, your capacity to change will be higher. If most of your factors are in the right column, your capacity to change will be lower. If they are a combination of both, your capacity will be somewhere in the middle!

Back to that change you were thinking of. Ask yourself, *how high is my change capacity?* If your answer is "not great" then it is going to be much harder for you to make this change.

Factors that Increase Capacity	Factors that Decrease Capacity
Younger age <35	Older age >35
Refreshing sleep	Poor quality or quantity of sleep
Cardiovascular fitness high	Unfit
Good mood	Anxiety or depression
Eat healthy food	Eat processed food
Non-stressful job	Stressful job
Job with regular hours	Shift work, especially with night shifts
Work hours < 40 per week	Work hours > 40 per week
Normal weight	Overweight
Steady weight	Dieting
No chronic disease	Chronic disease
No regular medications	Regular prescribed medications
No recent deconditioning event	Deconditioning event(s)
Non-smoker	Smoker
Control over your daily physical load	No control over your physical load
Control over your recovery time	No control over your recovery time
Good support Network	No support

Table 2 – Change capacity table

How Keeping a Journal Can Help

Asking the above three questions will hopefully help you to choose a change that is easier for you to make. To answer these questions requires you getting to know yourself better. It is not enough to know how change happens, you also need to explore your current habit flywheels and your change capacity factors. You can start to think about *how YOU change!*

There are eight billion people on the planet, but there is only one you!

The principles of change are common to us all but how you change is unique to you. The best way to see patterns in your life and gain a better understanding of what you are like is to observe yourself. "Follow yourself" on social media! Getting to know yourself can be made easier by recording your activities, your food intake, your weight, and/or your energy levels throughout the next few days and months.

In the clinic, I make a quick assessment based on the medical record of the patient and a short chat. I have spent years learning to spot patterns in this consultation. I am really trying to judge, based on my experience, how this person is likely to behave. I then customise the approach for each individual.

Your medical record is really a journal. Journaling is one of the most powerful things you can do when you are changing something. When we do something habitually, we often don't notice how often we do it or notice the details. If journaling seems a bit dull, get creative. If you have a phone with a camera on it, take pictures of everything you do for a couple of weeks, and you will have an instant journal. I did it and wow did I eat a lot of cheese! Figure out a journaling style that works for you.

While you are thinking about what you could change, perhaps just go nuts and spend a couple of weeks recording yourself like a social media star or an influencer. Get to know you!

Have Reasonable, Optimistic Expectations

You want to make a positive change in your life. It is very important to choose something that gives you a realistic chance of success. Think about the chefs who win the cookery competition shows!

It all depends on what you are trying to achieve.

Your body requires resources and time to change, and it's easy to overwhelm your body's capacity. By choosing a realistic habit to change you can ensure your body has the resources to adapt to the new information you're feeding it and allow for the habit to stick. The effect of one positive change often leads to other unexpected improvements as well. For example, exercise doesn't just improve your fitness but makes your mood better too!

If you still don't know where to start, there is one thing that will make the most of where you are now. Start to do more physical activity to increase your body's overall capacity. More fitness means you can do more of everything and that includes change! I will talk more about fitness in the coming chapters.

Do not be afraid of failure. Failure is an integral and essential part of change. How can you get stronger at the gym if you don't struggle to lift the weights? You can't learn to ride a bike without falling off, you can't learn to play the piano without hitting the wrong keys. You can't make any change without an element of overload that can be considered failure. The bigger the change, the more you are likely to fail at first.

Embrace failure as an essential part of change and keep going.

Finally, spend some time thinking about how to improve your *change capacity* by considering the factors in the change capacity table. Maybe add some factors you observe in yourself. It is impossible to change some of the factors (your age, for example), but think about those factors in the right column that you could shift towards the left. How can you improve your overall change capacity? Don't forget these are changes too!

The first stage of planning is choosing what you want to achieve and what resources are available to make that change. Having learned about how big the change is and your capacity for change, you should have a better idea of how much effort a particular change may take. Now you can choose something to change that you think is achievable. As you have read through this chapter, this will probably not be the original change you had in mind.

Next, we will look at a practical strategy to help you make this change. In the following chapter we are going to work on creating a plan and putting your plan into action!

Chapter 26

PUTTING YOUR PLAN INTO ACTION

Why is change so %#$*ing difficult?

Change can be hard because our bodies are efficient and the most efficient thing for them to do is not change. Sometimes we really do feel like we are fighting against our bodies, especially as we start to suffer the consequences of the long-forgotten choices we have made. However, there comes a time when we all need to change, either to do something we want to do or minimise the consequences of what we are doing.

Staying home is easier. Bilbo, in The Hobbit, would have preferred to stay home and not go on his "unexpected journey." He told his nephew:

"It's a dangerous business, Frodo, going out your door. You step onto the road, and if you don't keep your feet, there's no knowing where you might be swept off to."

Changing a habit is a journey. Navigating to your "change destination" can be a bit of an adventure, as it's easy to get lost. Now that you have chosen a realistic change destination with the resources you have available, you need a plan to get there. When you go on an adventure a map can be useful.

Gandalf made a plan using a treasure map that guided Bilbo on his adventure. In this chapter, I'll give you a "change map" based on five stages of change adapted from teachings by Noel Burch of Gordon Training International. He had only four stages; I've made a change by adding a fifth one!

To illustrate these five stages, I will draw on my personal weight loss journey. I figure that now I've kept my weight off for more than five years, I'm entitled to write a book about it! In all seriousness, *do not copy me*. My solution will not work for everyone, because my struggles and solutions are *unique to me*. However, learn from my adventure as I navigated these stages of change, tried out different solutions, failed, and committed myself to the one that worked for me. There is a solution out there that will work for you.

Stage 1: Unconsciously Incompetent (Not Knowing What You Don't Know)

Just as it can be hard to admit you are lost, many journeys of change begin with the hard realisation that you are unconsciously incompetent. This is when you are "clueless" and you don't know what you don't know. Ignorance is bliss. You are unaware that you have a problem. Many people are stuck in this stage for a very long time.

A few years ago, I was a busy physician doing lots of emergency room calls. I also had a busy, rural, family practice. My wife and I had four boys in under five years. I was stressed, tired, and hungry. Amongst all this busy-ness and chaos, I still considered myself to be a reasonably good, healthy example for my patients.

One day I saw a photo of myself sitting next to a swimming pool. What I saw in the photo did not match the version of me in my head. I hadn't noticed that I had been steadily gaining weight. I had been unconsciously incompetent of the changes happening in my body for many years. Until I saw that photo.

Stage 2: Consciously Incompetent (Knowing What You Don't Know)

At this stage the penny drops. You come to the realization that something is wrong. There are many things that may trigger this realisation. For example, you may experience pain, visit the doctor, or learn something you did not know before. You may read something or watch a video that turns a lightbulb on. At this stage you can start quantifying what is wrong and decide you want to fix it … you just don't know how to yet.

When I saw the swimming pool photo, I realized something had gone wrong. Like a good family doctor, I weighed myself, calculated my BMI, and congratulated myself on making the obese category.

No matter. I wasn't too concerned. After all, I was trained to deal with this exact situation. Without any thinking I put my plan into action. I pulled out my trusty rowing machine and started rowing. I had been a keen rower in my younger days so I knew how to get fit and shed a few pounds, *or so I thought*. After a few weeks of rowing, I weighed myself again and was surprised to see I was heavier! I did feel better in myself though. I was not as out of breath when I chased after my kids. My body capacity had gone up, but my weight had also gone up, and this was really annoying. For those who are having a similar experience, my best advice is not to start where I did! I made the classic mistake of making weight loss my first goal rather than increasing my body's fitness.

It was at this point that, despite all my years of medical training, I realized I was incompetent. My go-to plan of hitting the gym had not worked. I recalled a lecturer saying, "All you need to know is that energy in equals energy out, plus fat!" *Easy*, I thought. More energy out meant less fat, but muscles weigh *more* than fat. I figured the weight gain was because I had gained more muscle than I had lost fat. All I had to do was exercise *more*.

A few weeks later, I checked the scales again. Annoyingly, forty-five minutes of working out two or three times a week was not having the expected results. Now I knew for sure I was incompetent. I needed a better plan. In the end, I had to embrace the unacceptable "f" word. I had failed.

Stage 3: Consciously Competent (Knowing What to Do)

With some research you work out a plan and start to become more successful. You understand what is wrong and come up with a strategy that works for you. You start to put your plan into action, a habit starts to gain momentum. Some failure is normal at this stage. You can't make a new, dominant habit without occasionally falling back into old, well-established ones. The old habit flywheel can take a long, long time to spin down. The new one can take some time to spin up. Expect and accept some failure as part of change.

It was time to stop and take stock. Coming up with a better plan needed some preparation. To lose the extra weight, I first had to quantify the problem. I spent a few weeks writing down and taking photos of everything I ate. I was honest and just ate normally. Next, I looked at what I ate a lot of. It turned out to be cheese and chips. From tracking my eating habits, I saw how often I snacked in the evenings and decided that cutting down on that would be the answer.

I felt strong in my resolve and cut down on my snacking, but I was miserable, hungry, and exhausted every evening. Lack of sleep and the continued stress in my life made me crave my snacks. I slipped back into my old habits. In the end, I talked to my wife, and she said she could lend a hand. I reluctantly admitted I needed help.

One day I went to the fridge and found small bags of cut-up cheese. In the cupboard there were lovingly prepared snack bags of chips. It seemed like a lot of effort to put such small amounts of food into bags for our children. I asked my wife what she was up to, and she said she had read that putting snacks into 100-calorie portions helps you see how much energy is in them. This helped me snack in smaller portions! It turns out it doesn't take much cheese to make 100 calories.

After a few days, some larger bags of sugar snap peas and carrots appeared. My wife said, "Now you have a choice. Each bag has roughly 100 calories in it. You choose."

*"What do you think I am, a ****ing rabbit?"* I silently protested.

For the first time in my life, I realized how little I knew about food. It was time to do more research. A brief investigation convinced me to start snacking on the "stuff" in the larger bags.

Up to that point, I had considered a vegetable as something to accompany a steak or to dip in mayonnaise, but after a few weeks, I found I was enjoying the vegetable bags *more*. I was surprised the next time I stood on the scales. For the first time in a decade, I was not only aware of my weight, but it had gone down. I now had a plan that was working!

Slowly over the following weeks, months, and years, I read about food. What was working for me was hardly unique but what I learned was the pointlessness of following anyone else's plan. All diet plans succeed *if you stick to them!* Why we don't stick to them was a question that I didn't have an answer for.

This was the starting point of me asking the bigger question, "How does my body actually work?" This book documents the answers I came up with. I can now explain why most diet plans fail: They often don't address our unique and strong, individual, food preferences and our food-based coping mechanisms. Our childhood-developed food habit flywheel is one of the fastest spinning and heaviest we have. I realised that the food we eat has a massive habit momentum! This is why over 99 per cent of diets fail within five years. Not only do diets fail but the blame for your failure is directed at you for not sticking to the plan!

I made the connection earlier in the book between money and fat because your body's currency for life is fat! If you want to make a change in your spending habits, keeping an honest account of where you spend money obviously takes more work than just hoping your spending is ok. The same goes for tracking eating habits, but the extra work is well worth the effort. Your friend's dessert is not free of calories! It helps to be honest with yourself.

At last, I had found a strategy that was working for me, and I had become consciously competent. I had a good plan and could stick to it.

Stage 4: Unconsciously Competent (Having a New Habit)

After several months (and sometimes years) of hard work, you have made a change that has stuck. You no longer have to think about your new lifestyle or habits, as it is now hard-wired learned behaviour. You have a new habit! At this stage, you have successfully changed to address the original problem.

During the first few months of eating food thoughtfully, I learned a lot about the food I was eating. I learned how much food I needed, and what food upset my stomach (I used to ignore it and carry on, not understanding why my digestive system was so upset.) I had no idea that years of reflux and abdominal discomfort were due to eating wheat! Our family called it the "Barnsdale belly," and the smells from the farts produced could clear a room. I had tested negative for celiac disease in the past and had concluded that wheat wasn't the problem. After using a journal, I worked out that if I ate a hot dog, I would have pain within twenty minutes. Later in the day, other people around me would regret my decision too. Losing some unwanted weight led to some other beneficial discoveries too!

I am now years down the road. I generally know what food will make me feel good and what food will upset me. Making food decisions is now more automatic than when I was consciously competent. When I run into a problem, I have a strategy to put it right and it doesn't take much effort to implement it.

One of the most important things I learned was that I gain weight in an episodic way, in short bouts of overeating, rather than steadily over time. Because of this knowledge, I plan for Christmas, birthdays, and other holidays where food is a key element. I try to lose some weight before these events and plan for a "restoration" period afterwards.

I no longer see weight gain as failure because it is no longer out of my control or understanding.

I now embrace some episodic weight gain as part of successfully celebrating or relaxing on holiday. The journey, however, is never over, there is always more to know.

Stage 5: Maintenance

It is important that you maintain your change and reassess as you go. Continue to be aware that it is easy to slip back into old, well-established habits and be open to different ways of doing things. There is nothing in life that you can't continually improve on, even if you are writing the book on it! Be prepared to go back to Stage 1, if you need to.

For me, my struggle to lose weight opened my eyes to a greater hole in my knowledge. As a doctor, how could I understand so little about the operating principles of the body? I owned one and didn't know how to use it properly!

When I started to understand that the body's main operating principle is efficiency, it led me to look at the problem of weight loss in a different way. Using this principle to evaluate weight-loss strategies led me try intermittent fasting. (Go back to Chapter 22 to learn more about this strategy). If I need to lose weight these days, I focus on intermittent fasting, which works well for me. My wife does not have to fill those little bags full of snacks. Generally, my food habits are better (although from time to time my wife subtly "helps me" and the bags reappear – back to Stage 1).

Looking at what I ate convinced me of how unconsciously incompetent I was about food in general. As I learned more, I decided to try more "healthy" whole foods. Not only did I discover all sorts of new culinary delights but along the way learnt that as eating healthy food hurts you less, it can help you feel better. I still love a good steak, but weirdly for me, now I often enjoy the accompanying salad or vegetables more. I even spent a couple of months seeing how it felt to be vegetarian (the younger me just fainted in disbelief). I find the healthier I eat, the better I feel. Darn it.

I keep learning more about my body. In five or ten years' time, I may be doing something different. Life is a journey of continual change.

The Importance of a Good Story

Having a good story to convince yourself that you need to change and guide you in how to change is very important. The motivation for writing this book was to share some anecdotes that you can use to help you work on your own stories. When you have a good story to tell yourself, it helps you tag the "memory triad" with a positive "attitude trigger" that facilitates building up "habit momentum." I think I just crossed the line between acceptable jargon and BS. Translation:

We all like a good story.

You can now use the change map I outlined in this chapter to help you come up with a plan to successfully take you to your chosen habit destination. Just like Bilbo, I hope that this sometimes challenging adventure ends with some treasure and a good story to tell.

Chapter 27

MAKING A CHANGE – THE IMPORTANCE OF YOUR ATTITUDE

"The problem is not the problem. The problem is your attitude about the problem."

—Captain Jack Sparrow

Your attitude is hugely important if you want to successfully change. A positive, realistic attitude is much more likely to result in a successful change than a negative or unrealistic one. Your body wants you to be the best you can be. Why not work with your body? You could adopt the same attitude your body has: You are important and valuable!

During my weight loss journey, I learned how important attitude is, no matter what change you are seeking to make. I eventually realised that my attitude of "knowing it all" and "not needing any help" was holding me back. I also realised that an impatient, fix-it-now attitude was not helping either. Unfortunately, the quick-fix approach we so often hear sets us up for failure. Getting caught in a cycle of early success followed by hitting a wall is $%&*@+ annoying! Repeated failed diet plans can result in an attitude towards any healthy lifestyle choice as being a complete waste of time. It is easy to become discouraged and give up, but hopefully now you have the tools to figure out your own plan that will be successful. Patience will also help!

Working things out for yourself is the key to success. Abdicating responsibility to the latest media-inspired health fad is much less likely to be successful. Don't allow other people to lead you into another failure and worse than that, take your money whilst they are doing it. Take responsibility for your own journey. You are important! Your body certainly thinks so.

The best way or the easiest way? The two are often not the same thing. In the medications chapter, we talked about the difference between taking a sleeping pill to sleep versus learning how to get regular, unmedicated sleep. If your attitude to the problem is finding the best way, for the greatest long-term gain, you are more likely to be successful.

While taking ownership of your problems is important, you do not have to do this alone. It can be hard to admit you need help that goes beyond the latest self-help book or podcast. Asking for help is not a sign of weakness but rather a sharing in the collective knowledge out there that can help you "be the best you, you can be." There are a lot of people ready to help you figure out what options you have, and which are best. Don't forget to ask them:

"Who are you and why should I listen to you?"

It is so much more fun to learn why they are making these suggestions than to simply follow them. Filter their explanations through the principles you have learned in this book about how your body works.

Being Realistic about Your Attitudes

Admitting how you feel about what you do requires some bravery. If you take pride in working hard or have people depend on you for money, taking a financial hit because work has become too much and you need to take a break to recover, is a brave decision to make. Facing up to what has been going wrong is also a difficult, but important, step to take. Your body is the most valuable machine you own. Often the things that are the most valuable in life take the most effort to maintain.

Changing your attitude to your body's overload and recovery is so important. Failure is a part of change. Pain is a part of change. Fatigue is a part of change. Framing those feelings of failure with the right attitude is empowering. Learning what your body is telling you is the key to this. "Wow, I know I had a good workout in the gym yesterday because I can still feel it today" is a good attitude toward your aching muscles.

Become an expert on you. Become such an expert that *you* could write a book on how to be just like you. This includes learning about what food and which activities best run your body, and what your attitudes to different habits are. Learn to gauge how quickly you recover. You are the only one who can figure this out and compile a set of guidelines to meet the unique needs of your body. Start mapping out what you are like. Think of it as writing a travel guide all about visiting you!

What Am I Trying to Achieve?

Life is a journey. Your body is the vehicle that carries you on the adventure. What runs your body most efficiently is not necessarily the most rewarding thing in terms of life experience. If that was the case, there would be no athletes, no doctors, no explorers, and no war heroes. It's important to make the most of your life, which can include pushing your body. Life is too short to not occasionally eat those hotdogs if you want to. It is also good to learn the consequences of your choices. No one is happy when I eat hotdogs! There is normally a twenty-minute gap between my wife saying, "You'll regret it," and me agreeing with her.

Preparation Is Everything

The chance of you getting hurt this weekend depends on what you have been up to prior to this weekend. "Weekend warriors" get hurt a lot because they may not have taken the weeks and months beforehand to build momentum in their "weekend warrior flywheel." When that inevitable overload event happens, it is relatively larger and has greater consequences. Try to work like your body by anticipating and preparing for the future.

Prepare well. Stay well.

I want to ski every year so months before the season starts, I start cross training exercises that adapt and prepare my body in readiness to ski. As I build up my skiing flywheel momentum, I know I am far less likely to have a catastrophic overload event when the ski season rolls around.

Changing Your Attitude

You can also prepare yourself by practicing your habits "virtually" in your mind before you do them. At the start of this book, I stated that "your body does not know what you want to do, it only knows what you do!" Interestingly though, your brain can run the programs virtually without actually doing the action.

This previsualization is a neat trick to help you to improve an action before you do it. A golfer will perform a virtual, perfect, "dry run" of their next shot resulting in them sinking the putt. A politician will mentally run through an inspiring delivery of their keynote speech before performing it. A surgeon is taught to run through the whole surgery in their head before doing it. A Formula One racing car driver imagines driving the perfect line on every turn on the racetrack before the race begins.

This is a very powerful tool to improve the program your body uses to run an action without doing the action. This is all part of planning to do an action. The more you practice virtually in your mind, the better you will be when it comes to actually doing that action.

The other neat thing you get to do every time you previsualize or virtually run an old habit program, is to change how you feel about that habit (memory). You can change your *attitude* to habits by running through them in your mind and "reinterpreting them" in a way you choose to. This is the basis of a lot of cognitive behavioural therapies. Professionals can help you to literally change how you feel about things! You can learn to do this on your own too. How quickly your attitude changes, of course, depends on how much habit momentum that attitude has. Change takes time.

Changing What You Can, Accepting What You Can't

Life is a game of numbers. It is a series of statistical chances, just like a game of cards. You can't always control the hand you have been dealt, but how you play it is up to you. Try to invest in the things that are important to you and avoid wasting valuable resources on things that are not. At the end of the day, you do not have control of everything, so concentrate on changing the things you can change and accepting the things you can't.

Listen to and take care of your body, whilst living life as "large" as you choose to.

"Hey dude, watch me ski off this ****ing cliff!"

When I ski, I know I could wreck a knee, hit a tree, or get totally frightcited and decide it's a good idea to ski off a cliff. That's part of the fun! I prepare my body as best I can but regardless of the risk, I choose to ski because I love it. Somehow it always goes better in the previsualization stage for me. I limp a little these days.

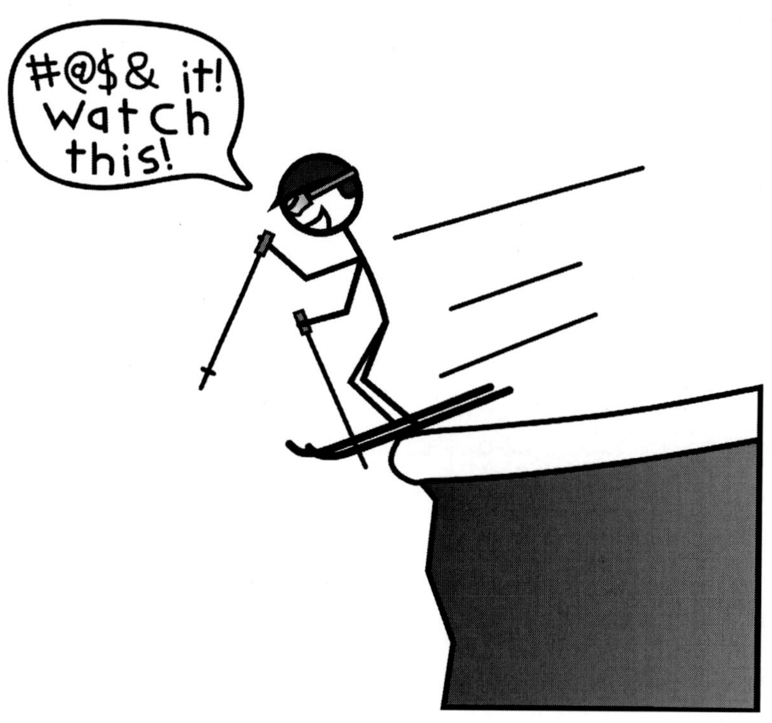
#@$& it! watch this!

Chapter 28

MAKING A CHANGE – QUITTING A BAD HABIT (LIKE SMOKING)

If you're wanting to make a positive change, you will inevitably uncover a habit that you feel like you would be better off not doing. A bad habit is something that has the potential to hurt you more than help you. Maybe your habit is obvious, like smoking, or less obvious, like snacking subconsciously on cheese every time you walk through the kitchen. No matter what it is, you probably want to change it.

Because I've talked enough about cheese and I'm not ready to give up the skiing, I will use the habit of smoking to illustrate the five stages of change through another lens. This will give you an idea of how to apply these five stages as you change an undesirable habit, whether that habit is smoking or something else. First, a little background on smoking.

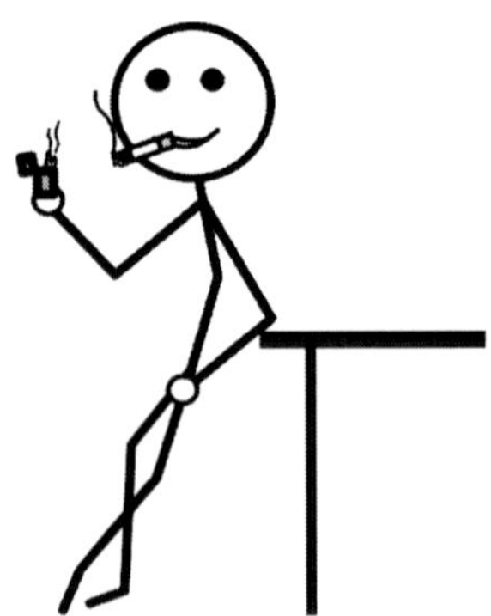

The Basics of Smoking

Cigarettes give your body a dose of nicotine, which is a chemical resource your body naturally produces to run some nerve cells. This drug (like all drugs) has an adaptive quality to it, which means that as you smoke more regularly and receive an added external source of nicotine, your hyper-efficient body will stop making its own version of nicotine very quickly. It's important to remember that your body will enthusiastically adapt to anything you choose to do consistently. If you choose to invest in smoking, your body will smoke to the best of its ability. There is a cost associated with the delivery of the nicotine as all the "nasty stuff" in the cigarette smoke can cause your body a lot of damage.

How Long Does It Take to Adapt to Smoking?

After only a few days of smoking, your body decommissions some of the machinery required to make its version of nicotine. This means that you quickly start to rely on cigarettes to provide your body with enough nicotine to function normally. You will get nicotine withdrawal if you skip a cigarette, which causes you to feel stressed and awful. Smoking another cigarette gives you the nicotine you lack and makes you feel normal again. Now, if you don't smoke you feel stressed! Some people start to smoke to manage their stress but do not realise that ironically it will cause them more stress than if they had never smoked.

How Long Does It Take to Re-Adapt after You Stop Smoking?

If you decide to stop smoking "cold turkey," it will take up to two weeks for your body to dust off and up-regulate its machinery to make more nicotine. However, if you slowly wean off cigarettes, it feels less jarring because your body can "catch up" and retool its nicotine-making machinery, starting to make nicotine while still receiving some from an external source. You will be less of a "&%$#" and be easier to live with if you do it slowly. If you still want to quit the cigarettes straight away, replacing the nicotine that you were getting from the cigarettes with nicotine patches or gum can help.

Habits for Your Habits

We have habits that support our habits. These supportive habits are not necessarily bad, they just subconsciously trigger our undesirable habit. You may not even realize what triggers your habit until you start monitoring your own behaviour. Don't forget that habits are just actions that are triggered by a part of a memory triad: an event, sensation, or emotion linked to that memory. We are quick to associate habits like smoking with other activities and routines like putting something in your mouth, waking up, or drinking coffee. These associations become automatic behaviours, making it harder to break a physical dependence. If you're a smoker, even reading some of these triggers may have caused you to take a smoke break.

Quitting Smoking: The Five Stages of Change

Stage 1: Unconsciously Incompetent (Not Knowing What You Don't Know)

There are many reasons to *start* smoking. It feels cool, rebellious, or grown up. It also may temporarily help with stress. As you become accustomed to smoking, it gives you a break from your routine. Realizing and admitting to yourself that smoking may be bad for you, and then deciding it is worth doing something about it, can be a big step. Ignorance is bliss. Unknown to you, smoking is hogging many of your body's resources because your body has to keep fixing the damage. You may be wondering why your injury isn't healing or why your illness is taking ages to fight off. Ignorance can also be deadly. The risk of dying from smoking is greater than nearly every extreme sport. Two out of three lifelong smokers will die from a smoking-related illness; it just doesn't happen as quickly as it would if you skied off that cliff.

Stage 2: Consciously Incompetent (Knowing What You Don't Know)

Like any habit you want to break, the first step after realizing there is a problem is to admit that you don't know the best course of action to address it. Today it's well known that smoking causes health complications, but this is still relatively recent. Only a few decades ago, governments and cigarette manufacturers refused to acknowledge the link between smoking and health problems.

The same happens on an individual level. Once you admit that the problem is in fact bigger than you've acknowledged in the past, you cross the threshold from unconsciously to consciously incompetent (Stage 1 to Stage 2). This is a great step; however, it's not enough to make a change. After all, many people smoke knowing it's not good for them.

To progress to the consciously competent stage, the smoker needs to decide that smoking is not worth the consequences. This can take a lot of persuading and regular encouragement from health care professionals, friends, and family. Many people who quit successfully have a story about a memorable event that changed their perspective. Maybe they lost a foot race to their eight-year-old because they were having trouble breathing, had an important conversation with their doctor, or learned that a young, fellow smoker at work was diagnosed with lung cancer. Many people only change a habit when they receive bad news about their health. The story of why you should stop smoking is very powerful. Remember that smoking is a huge investment of your body's resources that can stop you doing many things that you want to do. As an investment, it is like a million-dollar mortgage. You better love that house because you may not be able to afford to do other things.

Regardless of why you decide to change, the next step is to learn how to quit. There are many ways to stop smoking, and just like losing weight, something out there will work for you. Learn about different strategies and talk to people who have quit successfully to see if you have similar experiences and personalities. Try things on for size. For example, did you know there is a running club for smokers? As members get more serious about their training, it becomes easier to stop smoking.

The smoking habit flywheel momentum is often *extremely* high. Smoking can become the second most common thing that you do in your life! Breathing is something you do a dozen times a minute. This is going to be a big change! Prepare yourself and get help for this gargantuan challenge.

Stage 3: Consciously Competent (Knowing What to Do)

In the consciously competent stage, you have decided that smoking is not good for you and have started on a path to stop smoking. However, it will probably be very tempting to start again. Your body must re-adapt to not being a smoker. Smokers often initially feel terrible when they quit smoking as their body works hard to repair years of damage and to increase production of its version of nicotine again. Many people say, "I quit smoking and I feel like $#*%!" It may take your body a few weeks, or even months to finally get the chance to deal with all the crap that is lying at the bottom of your lungs. The feelings will pass, and you will soon feel better.

However, it's a good idea to have a *failure strategy*. A lot of people fail to quit smoking the first time. Choose a failure strategy that works for you. For example, you may have realized how much money you spent when you smoked. A good failure strategy would be to take out the cash you will save over the next few months by not smoking (based on past calculations) and buy something amazing for yourself. This way, you know you can afford it ... if you don't start your expensive habit again. Every time you feel like you want to smoke, look at the new car, the new television, or the photos of that holiday you already bought with your future cigarette money. Quitting smoking is the most important health choice you will ever make (and you'll be able to afford more cool stuff!)

Stopping any daily habit is hard. If you fail, don't give up. Try again or return to Stage 2 and use a different strategy. Remember that failure and change go hand in hand. One of the most important things you can do in life is

Learn to use failure to achieve what you want to do.

Stage 4: Unconsciously Competent (Having a New Habit)

Eventually, after not smoking for several months, you will start to think less about smoking. It takes several months to fully adapt to a new change. The more time that passes, the less you will think about smoking. One day, you won't think about it at all. You have finished adapting to not smoking.

Stage 5: Maintenance

Now that smoking is not part of your life, you can reassess things. You can even find something else fun to invest in! Smoking is riskier than hang gliding, so you now have many less risky options to consider.

Choose Good Coping Habits to Improve Your Life

You can apply the principles of change to any bad habit you want to try to quit. Bad habits are often coping mechanisms that we have learned to use to deal with difficult parts of our lives. It can be easy to simply replace one bad habit with another. Unfortunately smoking or vaping *anything* can be just as bad as smoking cigarettes. Switching cigarettes for another damaging habit is a wasted opportunity to improve your overall capacity. Instead, use the principle of efficiency to look for coping mechanisms that make your body work *better*. A good coping mechanism is an activity that helps you cope but also makes you feel better afterwards. It helps you more than it hurts you.

For example, exercise can help you cope with stress, improve your mood, and increase your body's capacity. Meanwhile, drinking alcohol can make you feel relaxed but at the expense of poisoning your body and giving it more to fix. It is usually easier to pour a glass of wine than go for a walk. Both exercise and drinking can help you to cope, but it is up to you to invest in your body deliberately. Again, there are a myriad of self-help books out there that promise you the solution to all of your problems. There is always some truth and value in other people's experiences. My advice is to listen to the advice but make it your own.

You are the best person to work on finding a unique solution for you!

Chapter 29

MAKING A CHANGE – INCREASING YOUR FITNESS

With so many things you could change, what will give you the "biggest bang for your buck"? There is overwhelming evidence that no matter what the problem is, getting fitter makes it better! If you asked me what you should change first, I would always suggest increasing your body's overall capacity, by increasing your fitness.

Some people enjoy going to the gym, but many of us do not. I personally do not enjoy getting hot and sweaty in a room full of other people whilst "pointlessly" lifting weights or going on a "virtual reality" bike ride that goes nowhere. Gyms are great if you enjoy them or have a purpose for lifting those weights. I prefer getting outside into the real world and getting some fresh air! Getting fitter is best done by choosing an activity you already enjoy that gets your heart pumping a bit harder. Walking a dog, joining a running or cycling group, or even dancing with friends could work better for you. Find something that you think is fun!

From Chapter 25, "Choosing a Change," remember that a good rule of thumb is that it is easier to work on something you already do rather than start something from scratch. Buying a brand-new piece of exercise equipment or signing up at a gym for the first time can be too much of a change.

Look at all the classified ads for rarely used steppers or bikes, or see how many people fail to show up again after their initial gym membership induction.

Upgrading Your Body's Overall Capacity

Here is how to use the five stages of change to upgrade your body's overall capacity by doing something active that you enjoy!

Stage 1: Unconsciously Incompetent (Not Knowing What You Don't Know)

The first stage is to realise the importance of fitness in your life and accept that you may need some help to learn how to do it well. Even if being active has been a big part of your life in the past, at this point in your life, you could still be incompetent!

Don't be put off by past bad experiences. You may have hurt yourself in the past, by doing too much for your body's capacity and not having adequate recovery time. As you've learned in this book, overtraining is a common problem in all areas of life. The benefits of exercise are so great, it is worth trying again. With help, you can find a new way to increase your fitness – you just may not have thought of how yet.

What you've been able to do in the past is a predictor of the future. However, don't forget that as you get older your capacity slowly decreases. More importantly, remember that when you stop an activity your habit flywheel winds down. For example, starting running where you left off five years ago could be a recipe for disaster. Running 1 km when you used to run 50 km seems pathetic, but you need to figure out what your body can do *today*!

Stage 2: Consciously Incompetent (Knowing What You Don't Know)

Before you start a new regime, remember it is wise to take a little time to figure out what will work best for you now. Do your research and choose an activity. Once you have chosen your new activity you can come up with a plan and put it into action.

The best way to change any activity is to introduce it gradually into your life. You can use your knowledge of the tear-and-repair cycle to train your musculoskeletal system, allowing for full repair between efforts. You need to slowly build on your range of movement and strength to adapt your body to do the new task. This takes time!

Listen to your body to decide how often to do your new activity, and how difficult to make it for yourself. Make observations as you go – how much is too much? It helps if you can quantify how much of the activity you do by recording time, repetitions, or your workout schedule. Learn how to *use aches and pains* as a gauge of how much of your capacity you have used or how far over capacity you have gone. Be cautious as you learn. When you start to ache and feel tired, this is a good time to stop.

Wait until your aching has returned down to the baseline (which may take a day or more) before doing the activity again. Also, listen to your emotions and how you feel. Do you feel recovered and ready to train again? Because you're consciously incompetent, you are truly in an observational phase, paying attention to how your body responds and adjusting as you need. As you continue doing the activity, you begin to understand your body more. How much you can repair can vary day by day, as your body calls on different resources. Your body will likely have other things to do and other system overloads to repair. Remember a glass of wine may help you unwind but it gives your body more to fix. Exercising the day after a big night out is not awesome.

As you slowly increase the exercise load (the length of time you do it, the repetitions, the weight, etc.) a good rule of thumb is to increase it by 10 per cent every two weeks. This is considered a safe interval, with minimum overload that can be repaired and upgraded within twenty-four hours. However, you can absolutely experiment with how fast you incrementally increase your exercise load. If you are aiming to improve faster than 10 per cent every two weeks, watch for signs that you are causing more damage than improvement. The emphasis should always be on recovery. Don't be tempted to go too far too fast, it really is counterproductive. Slow and steady wins the race.

Low and slow is the way to go.

In this figuring-out stage, consider getting expert help. Join a team of people who are more skilled and experienced, hire a personal trainer, or join a training program. Beware the young or inexperienced practitioner who may push you too far, too fast with promises of a quick fix. Tell them about this book! Experts are there to measure and witness your gains, and to watch for risk of injury, posture issues, or signs that you're doing too much. They essentially assess your body's ability to tear and repair and guide you as you increase the difficulty.

Stage 3: Consciously Competent (Knowing What to Do)

In the consciously incompetent stage (Stage 2), you learned your new activity enough to do it with more skill and confidence. Keep slowly increasing your activity until you reach the level you are aiming for. Listen to your body as you grow stronger and maintain your level of activity to maintain your capacity.

At this stage, it is easy to fall into the trap of thinking that as you become better at your chosen activity, you won't feel as much pain. It seems only fair that, by this stage, your pain after working hard should be improving. Annoyingly, this is not always the case.

How Do I Know That I Am Getting Better?

People often complain to me, "Physio does not work." They tell me that they went to a physiotherapist who gave them exercises and their pain got worse. It is frustrating when you try to improve something but the thing you are trying to improve actually feels *worse*.

> ***"Anything worth doing is worth doing badly."***
> ***—G.K. Chesterton***

Remember, you can't change anything without an element of failure. You can't build strong muscles without first tearing them and making them weaker. If you are chronically fatigued, when you exercise you will feel *more fatigued*. Confusingly, things seem to get worse before they get better. Don't give up. With enough time and dedication, and an emphasis on recovery, they do get better!

Overload makes the very thing you are trying to make better feel worse!

New Habit	Initial Bad Feelings	Functional Outcome
Strengthen your muscles	Your muscles ache and feel weak	You get stronger
Stop smoking	You want to smoke more and you feel grumpy as @#%&	You don't want to smoke
Change your eating habits to shed unwanted weight	You feel hungrier than ever (hangry)	You feel less hungry and also healthier
Exercise to boost your energy	You feel even more fatigued	You gain energy
Learn to play the piano	You hit wrong keys and people tell you to stop	Your skills improve and people recognize the tunes!
Save money	You feel frustrated because you can't buy everything you want	You have more money in your bank account and can buy that one thing you've always wanted
Ride a bike	You fall off your bike and scrape your shin	You can ride your bike
Improve your sleep routine (aka sleep hygiene)	You sleep less well and struggle to get up in the morning	You sleep better so feel less tired and recover more quickly

Table 3 – Confusing effects of change

When I have a frustrated patient, we go over the concept of "no pain, no gain, but don't overtrain" together. This is all well and good, but then they ask, "If I always feel pain when I work out, how do I know I'm getting better?"

The answer is to measure improvement with something other than pain! The concept of "functional" improvement is the key to judging your progress in all circumstances. No athlete can compete without pain. In fact, pain is the key to successful training. You can use pain to judge how hard to push when you are training and competing, and also to determine when you are recovered and ready to train again.

Athletes use pain as an "exertion gauge" to guide their effort as they train and compete. Athletes do not use pain to judge their overall performance.

To judge overall performance and progress, athletes use the measuring tape or the stopwatch. How well you are doing cannot always be measured by the level of your pain.

When I was a young man at Cambridge University, I joined my college's rowing club as an amateur. I had three years ahead of me and was keen to test my athletic prowess. After completing my first race, I was leaning over the side of the boat, trying not to puke and feeling like I was going to ****ing die. As I sat there feeling like $#*%, I told myself that I would train hard and in three years' time I would finish a race and feel ****ing awesome!

After three years of training and rowing in multiple competitions, I heroically completed my last race. As I sat in the boat at the end, trying not to puke and feeling like I wanted to ****ing die, I remembered what I had told myself three years earlier. I wondered what had gone wrong. I felt exactly the same way as I had at the end of my first race. This was all very disappointing. *Perhaps I'm just not a natural athlete*, I thought.

How could I work so hard for so long and feel like I failed? Now I know that I was judging my success in the wrong way, mistakenly using pain and fatigue as a measure of my overall performance.

If you take your body to the limit, it will always give you the same "you've reached the limit" feedback. If you run as hard as you can it will feel the same way, whether this is your first run ever or you are completing a sprint race after years of training. Pain is just telling you that you are going as hard as you can. The functional *measurements* of your overall performance tell you that *at your limit* you are improving.

Even though I felt the same pain after a rowing race with three years of training under my belt, I had improved a lot. Let's look at function. In our very first race, it took our boat twenty minutes to complete and it took me two full days to recover. After three years of training the same race took fifteen minutes and I recovered fast enough to race again later the same day. I rowed much faster and recovered much quicker.

This does not mean that your pain cannot improve over time. If after three years of training, I went back and rowed at the pace of my first ever race, I would have felt very different. I would miraculously have felt a lot less pain or none at all. Training for three years had elevated me to a level of functional capacity that meant that my novice race pace would have felt more like a warm-up.

Pain is present simply to tell you how your body is doing at this present moment in time. To get a better idea of how well you are doing, look at your *overall function* and *recovery* as outcomes, not pain. Think of it this way: *Olympic athletes and older people have a lot in common*, because they are both pushing the upper limits of what their bodies can do. The aim with fitness is to get your function to a level that allows you to do what you want to, with an acceptable level of pain. Don't forget, upper limits apply.

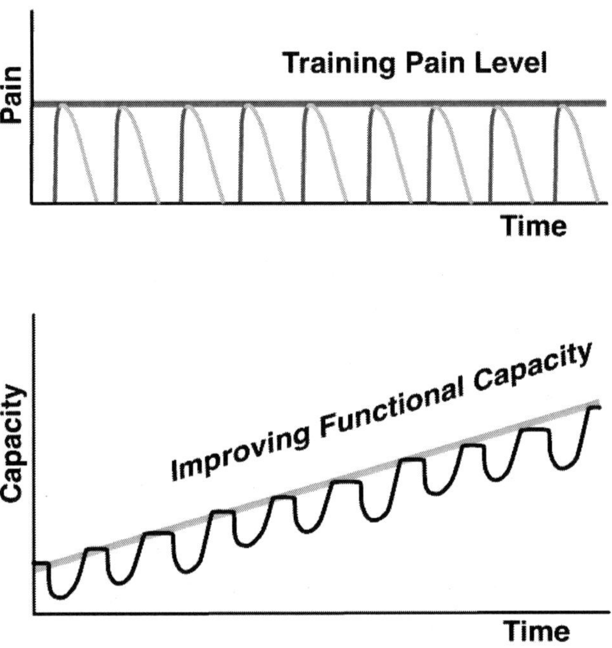

Improving function is a better outcome measure for success than pain.

Stage 4: Unconsciously Competent (Having a New Habit)

After several months, and sometimes years, of hard work, you have made a change. You no longer have to think about your new activity as it is now hard-wired, learned behaviour, and you are adapted to it. For example, three years ago you may have been incapable of cycling for five minutes without taking a break, but now you can cycle around all afternoon with your friends. Enjoy your new activity! If something changes, like if you get injured, go back to Stage 2 (you now have some re-learning and adapting to do!) and proceed from there.

Stage 5: Maintenance

Once you have increased your body's overall capacity by getting fitter, you can choose what you are going to do with your body's upgrade. Fitness allows you to do more of *everything*. In the maintenance stage, many possibilities are now open to you. You can think about ways to change your body to make it last longer. For example, now that you are fitter, you could start adding in some strength training. Increasing your strength may protect you from future injury.

Fitness allows you to do more. Strength is protective.

Whatever you do, make sure it is something you enjoy. Always keep an eye on your recovery and watch out for those deconditioning events! Take pleasure in being able to do more and recover more quickly. With an increased whole-body capacity you can now change anything more easily!

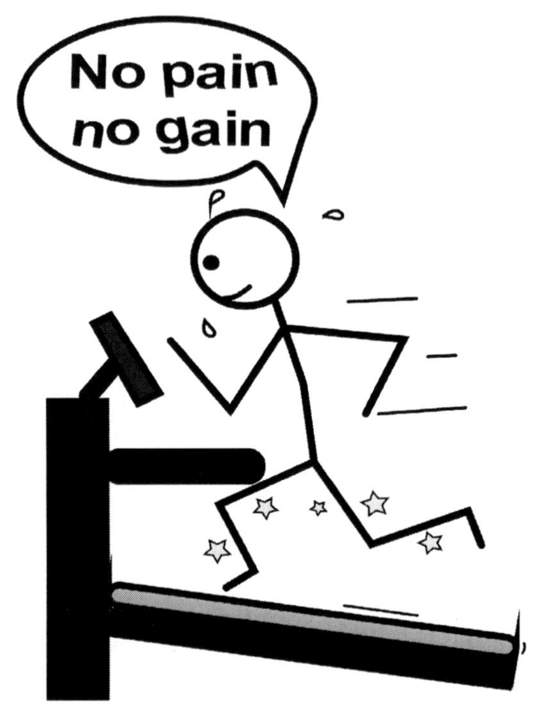
No pain
no gain

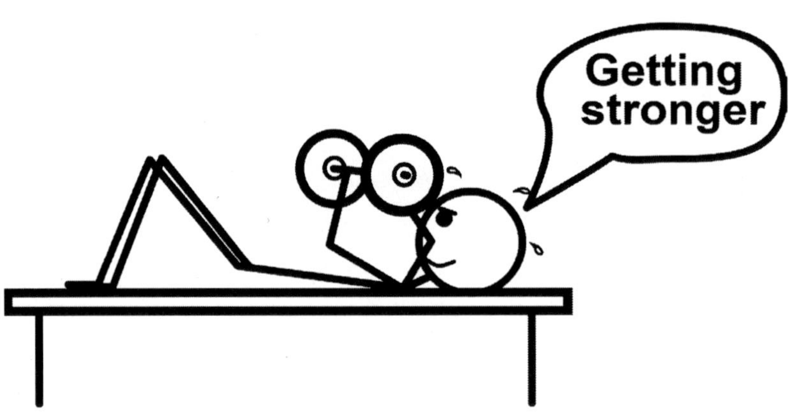
Getting
stronger

Chapter 30

MAKING A CHANGE – RECONDITIONING AFTER DECONDITIONING

You are nearly at the end of the book. Warning: This is a LONG chapter. This will be a test of your book-reading capacity! Before starting this chapter you may want to take a break or get yourself a snack, or if things are desperate, something a little stronger! (Like a cup of coffee ...)

Everybody knows that when you have an injury, you need to rest and give your body enough time to repair. When a repair takes many weeks though, it can feel really annoying, and it's easy to become impatient.

I don't have any magic to make your body heal faster, but I can tell you a thousand things you can do to make your body heal slower!

The most common thing people do that prevents the full healing of their injury is return to activity too quickly. That is, they don't allow their body enough time to complete Plan A. It can be frustrating, but healing takes time.

How Long Does It Take to Recover from an Injury?

Exactly how long it takes to recover depends on many

factors: how big your injury was, how high your capacity to heal is, and how much you can "let it heal."

Here are some general guidelines about how long recovery might take. The initial repairing phase (when it often hurts like $%&*) can take between two and fourteen days. Once the major overload symptoms (acute pain, redness, swelling, heat, and loss of function) have decreased, your body attempts to restore its basic function. This getting-back-to-basic-function process may take a further two to twelve weeks.

Once basic function is up and running again, your body can enter the "reconditioning" phase, which means strengthening. Getting back up towards your previous capacity can take anywhere from six weeks and six months. Once you have reconditioned, depending on how complete the repair has been, you have to retrain your habits to accommodate this new level of function. This retraining phase, of readapting your function to your new situation with a new capacity, can take from six weeks to five years! The whole recovery process from start to finish can take a long time.

Why Does Deconditioning Happen after an Injury?

The problem is that when you rest to allow your body to heal after an injury or during an illness, you will then become deconditioned. Remember the astronaut who deconditioned in space. Allowing an injury to repair inevitably involves some deconditioning. Once repair has finished then reconditioning may begin. In order to allow yourself to repair you lose some functional capacity, and that requires you to regain that function again afterwards. There is essentially a race between deconditioning and reconditioning.

It's important to note that it doesn't matter *why* you are deconditioned for this to hold true. You may have skied off a cliff and broken your leg or had a torn ligament surgically repaired. You might be in Plan B due to a tennis elbow injury (repetitive strain) from overusing your mouse, or maybe you were in a car crash that gave you whiplash putting you in Plan B+ (chronic pain) for years. Perhaps you retired from your physical job and stopped being so active, choosing to rest after a life of hard work. It could even be that a nasty virus has left you with chronic fatigue.

Osteoarthritis, a Common Cause of Deconditioning

Everybody, who lives long enough, gets worn knees, to some extent. Most people are not aware of the slow process of their knee joints wearing out and their capacity decreasing over time. Just like slowly getting wrinkles and grey hair, wear and tear happens to everyone (some more than others!). As they age, most people get some aching pain when they go for a long walk, but they naturally rest until it feels better. Since their pain goes away, they do not worry.

People with osteoarthritis pain that stops going away might end up in my clinic. This is the typical osteoarthritis story I hear: You go for a nice, long walk one day, walking further than you would normally. When you get back, your knees ache. After a night's rest, your knees feel better but are still aching. Your friend invites you on another long walk, and you decide to go along. Not far into the walk your knees start aching even more. You push through the pain to get home, and now your knees are really sore.

The next day, you go shopping and it feels painful to walk even the short distance around the store. The day after that, you go to a friend's birthday and stand in their backyard for the afternoon and your knees feel so terrible that you limp back to the car. After this episode, resting doesn't seem to help. Slowly the baseline level of pain you feel worsens. You have no idea what's going on.

What Is Going On in Osteoarthritis?

It does not matter how broken your body is, it will try to find a work-around to return you to the best function it can. For example, as your knee cartilage wears out it cannot be fully fixed, and eventually the cartilage wears down to the underlying bone. "Bone on bone" sounds bad! However, it is not as bad as you may think.

The good news is that your body always has another plan.

Your body thickens up the bones and they slowly remodel and adapt by changing into hard, smooth bone, a bit like ivory. This is not as good as cartilage, but it's not a bad second best. There are lots of people walking around with "ivory knees" who do not know they have worn-out knees!

However, osteoarthritis is the *pain* that results from overloading a joint that is wearing out (it has a decreasing capacity). Typically pain from overloading a joint is dull and aching, like a toothache, and generally gets worse with activity and better with rest. People commonly do one of two things because of this pain. They either use the joint less to avoid the pain, or they carry on and push through the pain.

Both actions can lead to deconditioning.

It is obvious why using the joint less leads to deconditioning. However, pushing through the pain can also cause deconditioning. This is because using your knees beyond their limited capacity all the time is overtraining, which means repetitively overloading without adequate repair. As you get older, overtraining is easy to do. We discussed this in Chapter 16.

What Can You Do about Deconditioning?

If your injury did not cause much deconditioning, simply go back to Chapter 29, which is all about increasing your fitness, because you are not in Plan B. If you are significantly deconditioned or in Plan B or B+ (chronic pain), read on.

The good news is that you can apply the upcoming five stages of change to recondition after any injury or deconditioning event. If you are in Plan B+ you can still use these reconditioning principles but you will probably need some extra help managing your pain while you do it. At the end of the chapter, we are going to talk what about to do if your pain is so bad that you simply can't do any activity, followed by what to do if that doesn't help, and you really need rescuing.

The Five Stages of Change to Recondition

Do not despair. It does not matter how broken you are or how long the problem has been going on, your body still wants to make you better even if your new capacity may never be as high as you would like. Much of my job is being a "grief counsellor" for people grieving their loss of function, whether it is due to injury or age. This is hard stuff!

However, you will not know what your new capacity is until you try. Usain Bolt, at one time the world's fastest sprinter, did not know how fast he could run until he trained his body. You do not know what your body can do or how well it can recover until you give it another go. The following five stages of change can be applied to improving Plan B pain, like osteoarthritis, in your knees. They can also be adapted and used to recondition any injury or deconditioning.

Stage 1: Unconsciously Incompetent (Not Knowing What You Don't Know)

In this stage of osteoarthritis, you spend each day pushing through the pain, trying to do basic tasks, and maybe taking over-the-counter pain medication to manage it. Sometimes, the episode that started your knee pain is now so far in the past that you've forgotten when or how the pain started. You want to walk but your knee pain comes on quickly and you can't go as far as you would like. The result is pain you do not understand.

If you have been injured like this, either suddenly or over time, you know how stressful, frustrating, and scary the experience can be. *What do I do?* You ask yourself. *Is this the way it's going to feel forever?* Thankfully you have this book, so hopefully this stage won't last much longer. The first thing to understand is that with any injury, your capacity to do *everything* has gone down. The second thing to understand is that you need to work at steadily regaining that capacity. Once you reach this level of understanding, you can move to the next stage.

Stage 2: Consciously Incompetent (Knowing What You Don't Know)

The pain in your knees gets bad enough that you decide to go to the doctor. There you get X-rays and learn that you have knee osteoarthritis. All you want is for the pain to go away and to be able to walk again. Depending on the factors that brought on your osteoarthritis and the circumstances in your life, you may be told to take some pills or lose weight. Likely, you will also be told to do some exercise, which seems counter-intuitive to you. Walking got you into this mess, so how can that help? Your doctor also tells you that your cartilage is wearing out or that your meniscus is torn. Such "catastrophic" language can make you want to give up.

Don't give up, there is a way to recondition your knees. When you are in Plan B or B+, the best way forward is to re-enter the faster Plan A tear-and-repair cycle. The following seven steps outline how to do this.

Step 1: Working out the baseline pain of your knees

When your body is in Plan B, it has started a chronic-inflammation program that may run in the background for months to years. If your pain has gone on for a long time, your body may have learned to report on pain and you will feel sensitized to that pain. At this point, you have entered Plan B+. Either way, this means you have a level of background pain that feels like it never goes away or comes on easily. This pain is not necessarily activity-related. This is your "background pain."

Choose a number from 1 to 10 that represents the level of the pain you feel all the time, your background pain. This number is your "baseline."

Step 2: Working out the capacity of your knees

This next step involves testing your knees. Now you have chosen a baseline number for your background pain, it's time to go for a walk. Make sure you have someone to follow you in their car, so you don't have to walk back in pain. Set a timer (or record the distance) as you begin your walk and stop walking when you have enough pain that you feel like stopping. Put a number on the pain you feel when you decide to stop. The time or distance represents the current capacity of your knees at this level of pain. For example, at ten minutes your knees might have gone from a background pain of 2 up to an uncomfortable 7.

Just like a weightlifter expresses his capacity by saying "I can bench press 185 lbs five times," the goal here is to quantify what your knees' capacity is. For example, "I can walk for ten minutes (or 1 km) before I feel like stopping with a pain level of 7."

Step 3: Working out how long it takes your knee to recover

After this walk, your regular baseline amount of pain will have increased because you pushed past your capacity. This is okay because you now have important information to work with. It's time to track something new: how long it takes for the pain to subside back to the baseline of pain you're familiar with. In other words, how long does it take for your knees to recover from this overload, back to what you're used to?

By asking this, you are really asking, how long is the healing program for this much walking?

If the healing program is twenty-four hours or less, you now know that you can repair your knees in that time. If you want to walk every day, it is important that you are fully repaired by the next day. Remember you only get the upgrade by completing the healing cycle.

Two things will tell you if you are ready to walk again. The first is that your pain number has gone back down to its baseline (in our example, a background pain of 2). The second is that you feel recovered and ready to walk again. If you feel tired or your knees are still aching at more than your background pain level of 2, do not go for a walk prematurely.

Step 4: Working out a safe place to start

When you feel recovered and your pain has returned to baseline, you can work out a safe capacity to start training at.

It can be helpful to quantify the distance you can walk and recover from in a day.

Calculate about 80 per cent of the time you spent walking, or 80 per cent of the distance you walked, as your starting point. If the first walk was ten minutes, this means planning a total of an eight-minute walk, the next day. If you calculated 1 km, this means planning a total of an 800 m walk. Split this time or distance in half as you will walk half the time/distance away and half of it back.

When you go for your walk away from your home and back (e.g., four minutes/400 m away and four minutes/400 m back) your knees will probably start to ache as you get home. This is okay! Your knees should start to feel better again the next day, because you didn't push them beyond your body's capacity to heal overnight. If your knees feel okay the next day, you can go for the same walk again.

Step 5: Fine-tuning your plan

If the ache does not return to baseline overnight or comes on quickly when you start to walk again, your knees are taking more than one night to finish healing. You also may not feel recovered. If this is the case, wait another day or two until your ache returns to the baseline pain you're accustomed to.

Working Out How Long it Takes to Repair

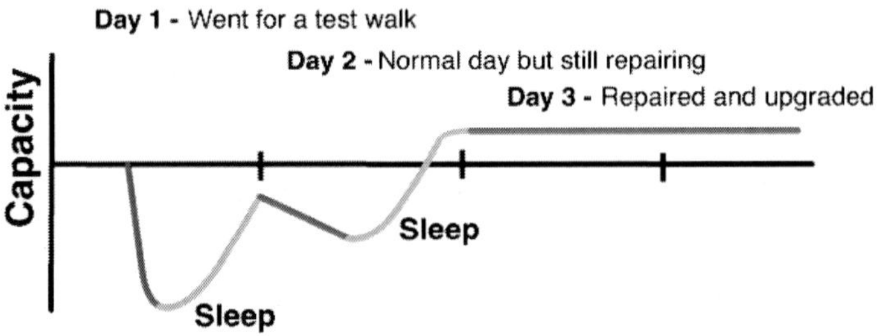

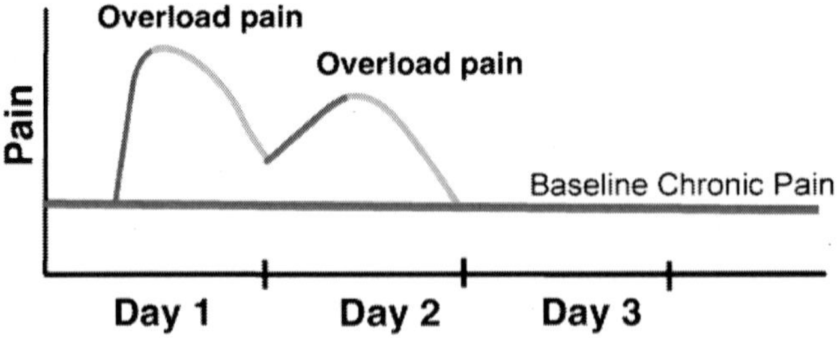

This is a sign that even 80 per cent is pushing it, so once your extra pain has subsided, decrease your walk time by around a third (e.g., from eight minutes to around a five-minute walk or 800 m to 500 m) and try again. If your knees still ache more than twenty-four hours after this walk, decrease it by another third, in this example giving you a total walking time of three minutes (one and half minutes out and one and half minutes back, or 150 m out and 150 m back).

The purpose here is to keep decreasing it until you find a length of time or distance you can walk that overloads your knees but allows them to repair within twenty-four hours. When you find this magic number, maintain it. You can then walk for this time or distance each day.

If You Want to Walk Every Day

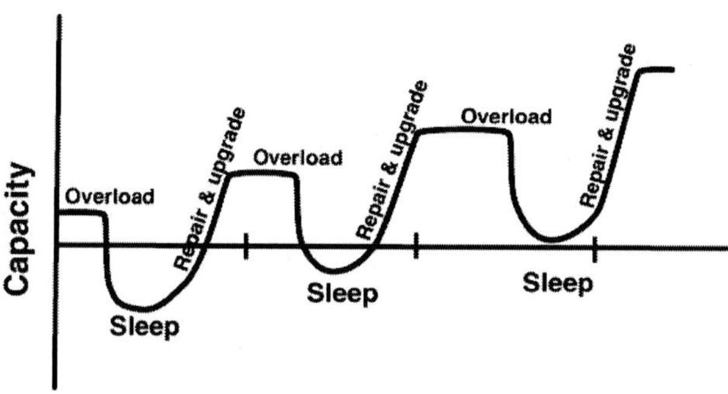

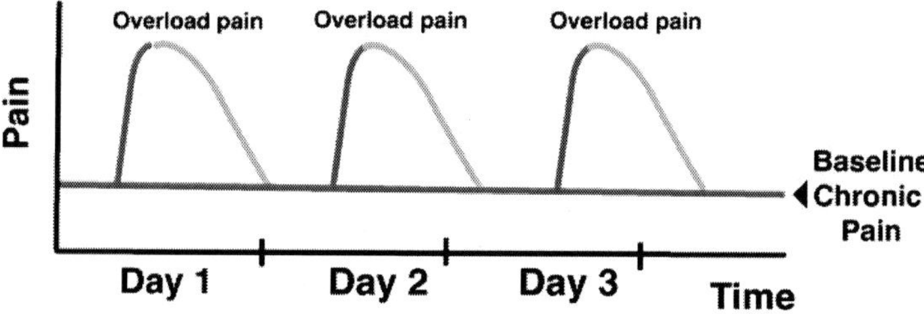

Step 6: Keep listening to your body

Not every day will necessarily be the same. You may wake up one morning and wonder why your knees haven't recovered like they normally do. Your body may be giving you a pain signal to tell you that it had to heal other things, as well as your knees, overnight. Your body can only heal so much. For example, if you had a nice evening and indulged in a few glasses of wine, your body will have had to fix the damaging effects of the alcohol on your body's other systems, so your knees will have had less of a share of the healing. Don't panic, just have a more restful day to let your knees catch up!

Pay attention to what your body is telling you. Don't forget that as you age your capacity will slowly drop, so keep an eye on how you are doing. Try to avoid thinking, *but I've always done this*. Ageing and wearing out are frustrating, so it's really helpful to get into the habit of listening to your body. Just because you recovered quickly last time does not mean you will this time.

Step 7: Slowly increase your load over time

When the walking is going well and you are consistently recovering overnight, consider increasing the distance/time you walk every two weeks or so by 10 per cent. For example, if you can walk for ten minutes, increase your walk time to eleven minutes after two weeks and note how your knees feel. If that goes well, after another two weeks increase it again by 10 per cent. The idea is to slowly increase your load with time. Don't be tempted to go too far, too fast.

This slow upgrade over time is the magic that can change your life.

This can be a slow game, and it isn't always a linear improvement. Keep monitoring your recovery, especially as you increase your load. Remember other factors in your life can affect your progress, like getting a cold or those glasses of wine you drank at the end of that glorious walk, and divert your body onto fixing something else and slowing the recovery of your knees. Slowly and carefully progress.

In the race of the tortoise and the hare, the tortoise wins.

Over time, this practice of minor overload and completed repair will increase your capacity. Your function will improve, and your aches will subside more quickly. Even the background pain (Plan B or Plan B+) may start to diminish or even go away. We discussed in Chapter 25 ("Choosing a Change") how change can have knock-on effects. The benefit of increasing your knee's capacity is that it will also increase your fitness. The more your knee can do, the more of everything you will be able to do.

Many people have worn-out knees but don't feel much discomfort, happily continuing the activities they love. They have increased and maintained their capacity to the point where they can do most of their activities of daily life. They intuitively rest when they overdo it. Most people who hear this story point out that this is just common sense! You too can get to this point by slowly reconditioning using the above steps.

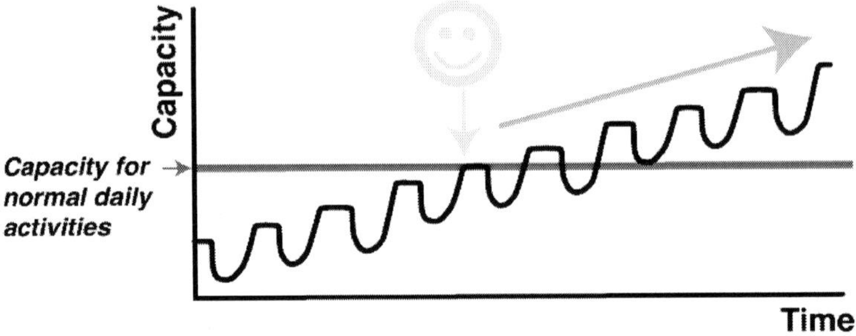

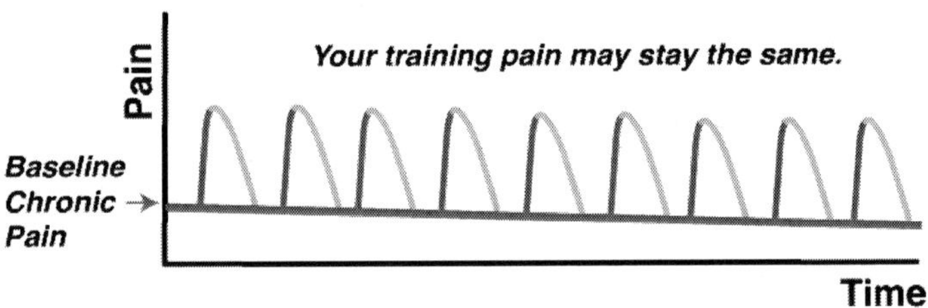

Once your capacity exceeds your daily needs your total daily pain will start to decrease.
Pain
Baseline Chronic Pain
Time

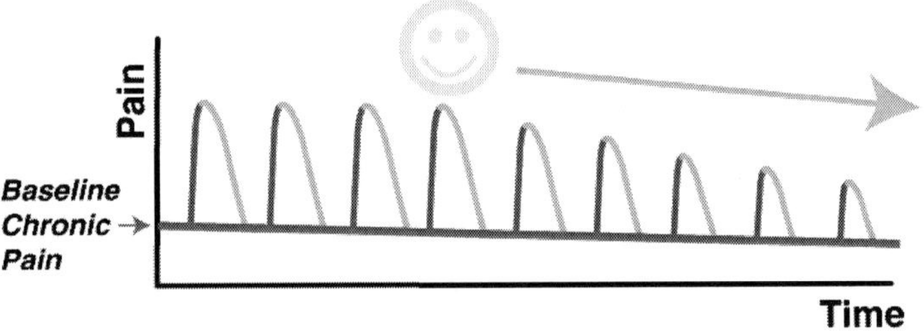

There are of course ways, other than walking, to train your knees. Some great ideas to consider are physio exercises, swimming, biking, ellipticals, and steppers. Find a way that works best for you and apply the same principles.

The consciously incompetent stage can be a difficult stage to navigate, but it can be made easier with professional guidance. No matter what your injury is, it is a great idea to see a physical therapist. They are personal trainers for broken people. They can help formulate a customised exercise regime that best suits you. While they can suggest how much exercise to do, remember that the only person who can judge your load and recovery is you!

Stage 3: Consciously Competent (Knowing What to Do)

Once you have learned how to use your tear-and-repair cycle to upgrade your knees, you are consciously competent! You have found that sweet spot between overload and recovery.

Movement is medicine and motion is lotion.

Remember the story of hitting your thumb with a hammer? If you hit your thumb and wake up the next day and it still hurts, the smartest thing to do is not hit it again! Few of us would take a pain pill so we could hit it again. The same applies to your knees. If your knee still aches, have a restful day. You may regret taking a pill and walking again anyway. That's what may have got you into trouble in the first place.

Stage 4: Unconsciously Competent (Having a New Habit)

After several months (or sometimes years) of consistent work, you have recovered. You understand your body well enough to deliberately stay within the capacity of your knees, and you know how to take the time to "upgrade" them. You now do this without even thinking about it.

Stage 5: Maintenance

Continue to do your exercises to maintain your capacity so you can do your activities. If you have another deconditioning event, go back to Stage 1. There is always more to any story and of course there is more to the story of osteoarthritis. As you work to maintain your function you may choose to find out more by reading books or finding an expert to consult. This may involve going back to Stage 2 "Consciously Incompetent" to do some more research.

Recondition Any Plan B Pain

I have shared the story of osteoarthritis, but you can apply the five stages of change to any deconditioning situation you find yourself in. The key to repairing any injury lies in making slow, consistent, incremental advances. Adjust the steps to fit your circumstances. For example, for chronic fatigue, instead of focusing on aching pain, focus on how tired an activity makes you feel and how long it takes to recover fully back to your original level of fatigue. Use the same principles outlined to adjust your activity level so that you recover before you want to do the activity again. Over time slowly increase your activity level and constantly monitor your recovery.

During any reconditioning process, it will sometimes seem like you are making things worse as you push your capacity beyond its current limits and feel the pain you normally try to avoid! Don't give up. Part of improving your function is pushing it. This discomfort is a crucial part of change. Also remember, that your emphasis should always be on recovery and your success is measured by your function not your pain. So, don't just sit there, make a plan! Get the help you need and, as we say in medicine, JFDI (just ****ing do it)!

If these reconditioning steps are working for you then you can now skip to the final chapter of the book. If despite your best reconditioning efforts things aren't going well, you may need more help, so keep reading. We will continue with advice for osteoarthritis, but the principles can work with other problems too.

What If You Can't Do the Reconditioning Steps?

What if your pain is so bad that you can't do any activity to recondition? There is still hope! Here are some strategies that you could try to make it easier for you to get moving and have a go at reconditioning.

Taking the load off: Because work done is "how far you can move a heavy object," this is a weight-bearing problem. Anything that can "offload the joint" can help control the load. Weight loss can help a lot, as every pound carried is multiplied at the knee up to seven times! You can carry a pebble a lot further than you can carry a boulder. Hiking poles or walking canes can take up to a quarter of the weight off each a leg. Use the pole or cane in the opposite hand to the injured limb so it acts like a "tripod" to spread the load. Sometimes special "offloader braces" can move the load onto a part of your knee that is not worn out. Decreasing the load can help with your walking capacity and recovery as you recondition.

Passive therapies: Most therapies that are not active exercise are considered passive therapies. These are treatments that therapists and doctors do to you. These help to manage your pain so that you can start your exercise to recondition.

Therapies can help with pain by manipulating the pain pathways, including medications, TENS machines, and injections, like cortisone. Other therapies are forms of injury that help kick the painful area back into the acute inflammatory cycle, Plan A. These include tissue massage therapies, needling, or joint manipulations. You may have heard of injections of hyaluronic acid or your own blood (such as platelet-rich plasma or PRP). These can also help with your pain in the short term to allow you to try to recondition.

What happens if you've tried everything, nothing works, and you're getting desperate? It's time to talk about surgery.

What Can You Do If Nothing Is Working?

If you have tried all the strategies to start reconditioning and have got nowhere, perhaps the time has come when you need rescuing; you may be past the point of no return. When you are in enough pain that it is stopping you from functioning, it is natural to want to be fixed, and soon! It is a big step, but surgery may be the only way forward. The only difference between surgery and assault with a deadly weapon is you signing a consent form. The skill of the surgeon is to injure you in a way that makes it favorable for your body to heal something that it cannot heal on its own. They could be chopping something out, tying something back together, or replacing something.

It's important to realise that it is not the surgery that fixes you, instead it is the changes your body can now make as it heals and adapts after this "skillful" injury. Once the doctor or therapist is happy that they have done what they can to make it favourable for your body to heal, the ball is back in your court! At the end of the day, it's all about "you fixing you." Time to try to slowly recondition!

Surgery is a big deal. Surgery is nearly always considered as a rescue or last resort. Not everyone with a worn-out joint needs surgery. It all comes down to your function.

When Do You Need Surgery for Osteoarthritis?

You may have been told that your X-ray shows that you are "bone on bone" and you need surgery. Don't forget though, there are lots of people in this situation who are doing just fine. If you ask the question, *Do I "need" surgery?* the answer is generally no. A comparison may help you to understand why a picture cannot predict function.

We already discussed that our bodies age with time. A photo may reveal wrinkles on your face. You could show that photo to a plastic surgeon and they could offer you a face lift. You may never have even thought about doing something so drastic about your wrinkles unless they were giving you a functional problem.

Not many people go as far as having plastic surgery. Not unless they have a functional reason to do it. For example, if you are a movie star and may not get that lucrative movie role, the pain and expense of plastic surgery may be worth it. Getting a face lift won't make you look young but pulling your skin tight behind your ears makes you look "Hollywood" and may be enough to get you that starring role. The same is true of your knee, you only need surgery if there is a functional reason to do it.

The best knee you've got is the knee you've got unless it hurts you!

However, if you are saying something like this: "I listened to your advice. I tried to lose weight. I tried getting fit and strengthening my knee with physio, walking, getting on my bike, aqua size, and swimming. I've tried walking poles, knee braces, and injections. I'm now taking pain pills every day. I can hardly walk a block. Nothing is working for me. You've got to do something for me, doc! My knee pain is wrecking my life!" The answer now to whether you need surgery is generally yes, you need a knee replacement.

If Surgery Is Recommended, What Do They Do?

In the case of osteoarthritis, there are a few options for surgery.

If only one part of your knee has worn out, sometimes the surgeon can break the bones to realign the knee to put load on the part that is not worn out, or just replace that one worn-out part. There are also new surgeries for younger people that try to patch up holes in the joint's cartilage.

If your function is bad enough – which generally means you are having trouble with your activities of daily life – a surgeon may offer you a knee "joint replacement." This is not a new knee, but an alternative made of metal and plastic. To put in the replacement knee, first they cut the ends off the bones and chuck them in the garbage. They then hammer on some metal to cover the ends of the bones and put a plastic spacer in between, giving you a metal-and-plastic knee joint. After this surgery you don't feel pain anymore because you simply don't have a knee joint that can hurt.

Unfortunately, this replacement also wears out over time. At this point you really do have something in common with your car! Your knee joint will no longer try to make itself stronger. How fast the metal and plastic wear out depends on how hard you are on it. Generally, the plastic lasts somewhere between six years (if you are a power lifter), and twenty or thirty years (if you are not). Once the surgeon has cut out your knee and replaced it with metal and plastic, it is crucial to heal around it and recondition because you just had a massive injury. Time to go back to Stage 1 and slowly recondition!

When Your Knee Pain Grabs and Stabs

With osteoarthritis, in addition to the aching pain, you may also experience stabbing pains or feelings that your knee is getting jammed or stuck, and your knee may give out when you feel these sharp pains. We call these stabbing pains "mechanical pains," as they represent something that is getting caught in your knee as it bends.

These stabbing pains are most commonly because of meniscal cushion tears. As knees wear out, at some point *everybody* tears their meniscal cushion although most do not even feel it. People who do get mechanical symptoms will find that they will normally go away within a few months as their body continues to repair, adapt, and remodel the knee. In this situation, the treatment is exactly the same as for aching arthritis pain: try to recondition!

If injections and reconditioning have not helped because those pesky bits of your meniscus are persistently jamming your knee on a daily basis or at worst a piece has got stuck and "locked the knee" so it won't straighten, you may need rescuing. In these situations, a surgeon will consider "cleaning up" your knee by trimming away and removing the bits of the meniscus cushion that are causing the trouble.

There may be some reluctance to do this surgery as your meniscus cushion helps to transfer load in your knee and cutting some of it away can speed up the wear and tear. Also, after surgery, your meniscus may tear again causing the stabbing pains to return. In the right circumstances this surgery can really help to get rid of those mechanical symptoms. After surgery, when your knee feels better, try to recondition!

Chronic Pain

As you have learned, every injury is an opportunity to get better. However, it's important to remember that if you are in chronic pain, the original injury may not be the problem anymore. Your body has done what it can, but you are left in pain. As your body is already oversensitive to injury, another injury (surgery) can make things worse. If you have a problem that has gone on for years and your doctor is not sure surgery will help, be certain you have tried everything else first. This pain is real and should be acknowledged, but it might be worth giving our heroic Plan A one last chance! It's time to try to recondition.

A Final Note on Buying "Snake Oil"

Seeking treatment for your musculoskeletal pain can be

very confusing. Just as there are many diet plans offering to help you lose weight, there are many practitioners offering to help you with your pain. The medical profession is more closely regulated than the dieting industry, so its claims tend to be less dramatic. However, there are lots of "alternative" therapies out there that offer to fix your pain. When you are in pain, you're an easy target because you are more open to trying anything that promises to take it away for good. Unfortunately, there are people out there willing to take your money and promise you a fix, even if their treatments don't do much.

As we have been discussing, anything that gets your body moving again and puts you into a completed Plan A cycle has the chance to make you better. If a practitioner tells you that wearing a daisy in your hair will make your pain better and you believe them, your experience of pain may change. Your attitude is very important. Remember, how you feel about your pain can change it. If you feel differently about your pain and start to move around more, you effectively give your body the opportunity to get better. Your practitioner will encourage you to attribute your improvement to the daisy in your hair, but the truth is that *Plan A is the magic that started to recondition your body*. If your practitioner can get half a dozen people to swear that daisies are the answer to your problem, then they have the start of a business. You could argue that there is no harm in this. It really depends on how expensive the treatment is for you.

This trick has been used for hundreds of years. In the wild west, travelling salesmen would sell cure-all snake oil to heal all kinds of maladies. So long as the treatment is not actually harmful, in the medical world we call this a "placebo." Placebos are "sham treatments" that aren't known to contribute to the healing of your body. Surprisingly, placebo treatments can work! If you believe you are going to get better, you may change how you feel about your pain. This is such a powerful effect that placebos can make people feel better up to around 40 per cent of the time. When you feel better, it's a chance to recondition!

The take-home message here is to be careful who you give your money to. There is no point in paying for something that your body can already do. It's a bit like owning a car but paying someone else to drive it for you. You are better off learning to drive your own car.

There Is Always Hope

Your body never gives up on you so don't give up on your body! This chapter could continue forever. We could discuss more and more problems and treatments that are available for your body. At the end of the day, it does not matter what the deconditioning event is, the answer is always going to be, try to recondition! If that does not work, try something else and then try to recondition!

"If at first, you don't succeed, try, try again."

—Old proverb

Chapter 31

MAKING THE MOST OF YOUR BODY FOR LIFE

What I've found in my career is that medical explanations are often full of complicated scientific language but offer little that really helps you understand why things are happening in your body. My hope is that this book has given you simple *principles*, in normal language, that help you understand your body so that you can make more informed, personalized decisions.

Making the most of your body involves having realistic expectations. Accepting that you are a biological machine that wears out will help you set more realistic expectations. You can use collective medical knowledge, gathered from years of observations, to help guide you as your body navigates its journey.

Life is a journey, and your body is the vehicle that carries you on this adventure. If you can understand your "vehicle," you can adjust your *expectations* according to the stage of the journey you are at. If you expect to have a fantastic meal while waiting to board at an airport gate, you are likely to be disappointed. A quick coffee and a tasty snack may be a more realistic expectation to help prevent a lot of stress. If you expect your body to do what it did when you were twenty-five years old, you may be just as disappointed.

***"Annual income twenty pounds,
annual expenditure nineteen and six,
result happiness.
Annual income twenty pounds,
annual expenditure twenty pounds ought and six,
result misery."***

—Charles Dickens, David Copperfield

It's all about "great expectations" ... Bad joke. If you spend less than you earn, life is easier. If you stay within your body's capacity your life will also be easier.

How Long Does Your Body Last?

Your body behaves a bit like a car in that it wears out over time. A human body tends to last around seventy to a hundred years, but systems can fail before this. In the same way that a car needs regular maintenance and repair to make it last, your body requires regular maintenance and repair to make it last! How well your body is made, how hard you work it, and how well you maintain and care for it, are all factors that predict how long it will last.

Most people think that a car wears out after it has done 160,000 km. Others think that a car can keep going to 500,000 km. A car that has driven 800,000 km is a rarity indeed! The truth is that there are different qualities of car out there. Different brands are associated with longevity, quality, speed, sportiness, luxury, etc. How well a car is made and how it is treated determines how long it will last. The same is true for our bodies.

If you consider a car as a collection of smaller machines or systems, this example still holds true. Each part has a capacity, beyond which it will fail. For example, brakes are generally good for around 50,000 km, and a battery typically lasts five years. If one part wears out prematurely, the car may be rendered useless, even if the rest of the car is in good shape. This can happen in our bodies too. If your heart stops, it doesn't matter how good a shape the rest of you is in.

What you choose to do is important. The way you choose to use your body, feed your body, and care for your body impacts how it specializes through adaptation. This is especially true when you are growing as a child. You can't go back and change what you did in childhood but if you are a parent, try to be deliberate in the habits you introduce your children to. Teach them the concepts in this book and help them to make their own informed choices.

When you become an adult, you start to wear out "unpredictably predictably," depending on how you use your body and how old you are. For comparison, if I give the same car to different people and come back twenty years later, the cars will be similar but different. If they use it as a race car, it will have a harder life and will wear parts out more quickly. If they use the car "normally" it will probably last longer. If they choose to store the car in a garage and never drive it, when they finally go to turn it on, it may not run well as parts will have deteriorated due to lack of use.

Just like a car mechanic has an idea of what may be wrong with your car based on its make, age, and use, your body's problems are predictable. Don't buy a used rally car if you want a reliable commuter! In the same way, if you have been a pro athlete, you may have some premature wear and tear in your musculoskeletal system. If you have spent years consuming a lot of processed sugar there is a good chance that one day you will be told you are now diabetic.

The main difference between you and a car is your ability to do your own maintenance and upgrades. If you want to maintain and upgrade your car, you take it to a garage. It won't repair itself – someone else must repair it. Cars are not adaptive. They do not "tear and repair" the amazing way your body does. The other difference between your body and a car is that you can replace a car when it breaks down and is rendered useless. You cannot replace your body. This means the stakes are higher! Your body is an investment. Invest wisely in things that are important to you.

Ageing Gracefully

The overall capacity of your body to do work slowly declines with increasing age. This is a fact that is rarely spoken about and is generally unpopular to bring up, especially when we're talking about middle age. The truth is that middle age is the time when we become aware of this decreasing capacity. Age and ambition always meet. Your body has crossed a threshold and simply cannot repair everything anymore. None of us are exceptions to this rule. We all experience this loss in different ways. We all grieve the loss of our youth and often start to reminisce about our "glory days."

This isn't awful news or a reason to throw in the towel on your effort to get stronger, in fact, quite the opposite. Many people continue to thrive at an impressive level as they age. Once fit in their twenties and early thirties, they keep active maybe hiking, biking, going to the gym, playing tennis, running, or skiing, over the decades. You meet them and can't help but notice how good they look for a fifty-, sixty-, seventy-, or eighty-year-old. They move with ease and grace, they are sharp in their minds, and have more energy than we're used to seeing in someone their age.

Even *these* people's muscles are slowly getting smaller and weaker over time despite their continued exercise. However, the fact of decline doesn't outshine the fact that they experience a much higher quality, more enjoyable, life; they get to travel, dance, and ski for years more than others. They sleep better, don't always get as much pain, maintain their independence, and experience fewer health complications. It's easy to hate these kinds of people! If you want to be one of them and are seeking the "Holy Grail," keeping fit is the closest thing we have.

I am often told that getting old is for the brave! If you understand your body, you don't have to be quite so brave. There can be a difficult adjustment period if expectations do not match with reality. If you embrace your decreasing capacity and modify your expectations, you can aim to age gracefully (or disgracefully, if you want).

One Final Story to End On

This is one of my favourite stories:

Brand-New Sports Car

We established that by the time you become an adult, your body has made its best guess during childhood as to what you want to do for the rest of your life. Your potentials are set. You are like a brand-new car driving off the showroom forecourt, able to quickly repair any damage to injury, working all day and partying all night, generally free of the fear of consequences.

Classic Sports Car

We talked about age and ambition meeting, which happens around thirty-five to forty, when most sports professionals retire as their accumulated injuries outweigh their ability to heal them. They simply can't keep up with the youngsters anymore. This is when you become like a classic sports car. This might be a difficult time as you adjust and grieve for the loss of your youth. As a "classic sports car," you can still do most of the things you could when you were younger but now if you "race," you expect the "car to be in the shop for some repairs."

Vintage Sports Car

As you continue to age you become like a vintage sports car. For most, this is in your fifties and sixties. At this point, you don't expect the car to race hard and if you tried, you would expect it to break. This does not mean you shouldn't drive your car. In fact, as sports cars age, people tend to love them more and their sentimental value, and even financial value, increases.

Antique Sports Car

You become like an antique sports car when your activities in daily life start to become limited. Generally, between sixty-five to seventy-five, age can really catch up with you. The consequences of long-forgotten injuries now start to affect your daily life. You need more care and attention. You can still do some of the things you love but at a lower intensity. Injury is much more likely, and recovery is even slower.

In the "antique sports car" stage you are more accepting that things are wearing out. You remember your glory days with fondness. If things go really wrong, this can be a difficult time. You must adjust to accepting more help than you are used to having. You have to learn how to get the most out of your ageing machine.

The trick is to listen to your body and match your expectations to your body's capacity during each phase. You don't always deserve the things that happen to you in your life. The best way to proceed is to accept the way things are and make the best of them. You can only change what is happening to you today.

"Yesterday is history,
tomorrow is a mystery,
but today is a gift,
that is why it is called the present."
—Master Oogway, Kung Fu Panda and others

Life isn't always predictable or fair. Never forget your body is on your side and wants to do its best for you. The most effective way to deal with change is to embrace it! Life is an adventure. Enjoy the journey!

In Conclusion

You picked up this book to learn why *Every Body Hurts*. I hope you now know it is because your body wants to help you be the best you can be. Consider this your invitation to begin improving some aspect of your life, starting today.

Your body will continue to adapt and change for the whole of your journey, helping you to thrive and function the best you can, with the "cards you have been dealt." Whatever has happened to you in the past, or will happen in the future, you will always have the chance to improve. Remember that your body loves you, it does not hate you! It is trying to give you what you want. Listen to your body. Learn its language. Pay attention to what it has to say. It tells you everything you need to know:

***"No pain, no gain,
but don't overtrain."***

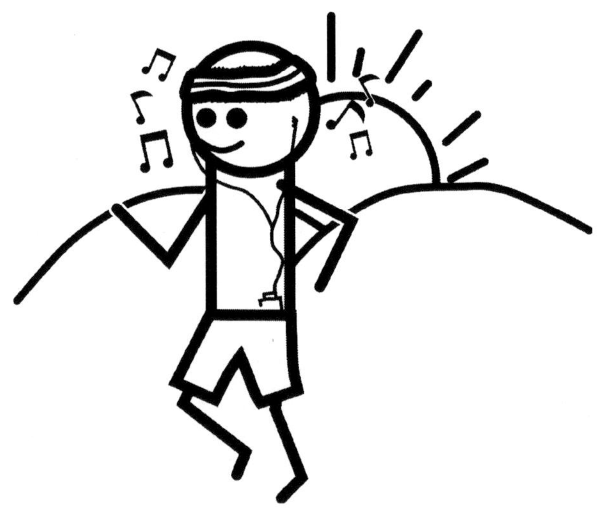

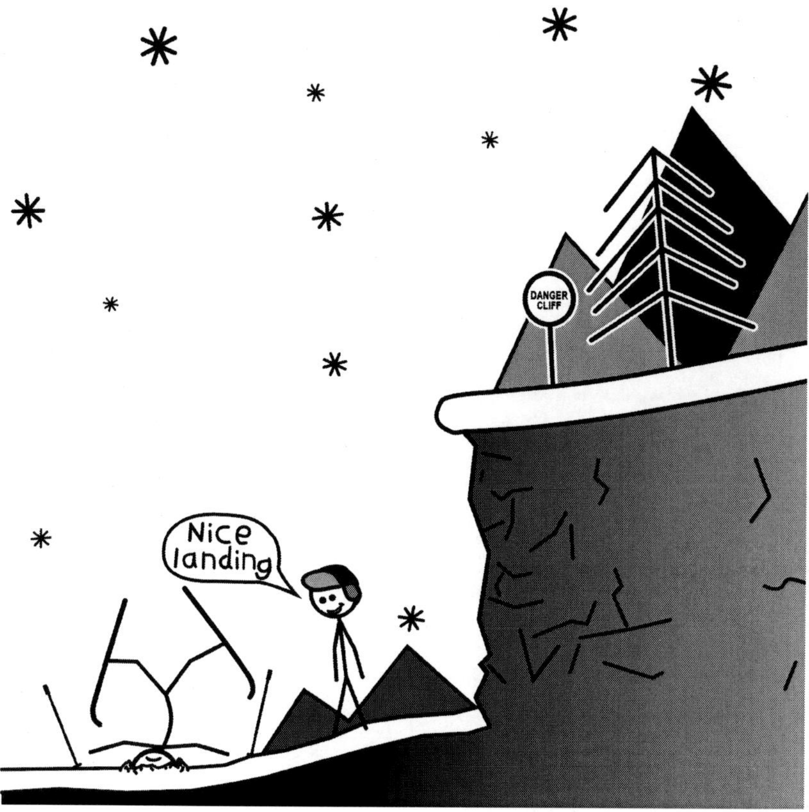
DANGER
CLIFF
Nice
landing

WHAT'S IN A NAME?

One constant in life is change. This book has changed a lot over the years, and I want to briefly share the iterations of the title that mirrored this journey.

Understanding Your Human Machine. A tomb of a textbook, coming in at over 100,000 words. Five long years of my life. Confusing. Long. Dull.

How to Change and Other Questions That Stump Doctors. Shorter. Great content. Less befuddling. Still disjointed and definitely not a publishable book. This is the text that went through the "Britt Machine."

Listen to Your Body, It Tells You Everything You Need to Know. True, but the title was too obscure. Vetoed soundly by Britt.

How 2 Upgrade U: Stories from a Doctor's Office. I was getting closer but again it did not capture the whole book.

**No Pain, No Gain. How the #$% Does That Work?** Blatant swearing is entertaining, and my office voted for this one. On reflection, not the right #$%ing title.

Why the #$% Am I in Pain? This is what my patients say to me every day. I am not sweary enough to carry this off in an interview though.

Every Body Hurts: A Physician's Guide to Making the Most of Yours. Punny. Thank you, Steve. You nailed it. I wish I had come up with it myself. We all need help!

ACKNOWLEDGEMENTS

Writing a book is not as easy as it appears. I have a whole new appreciation for the gargantuan effort it takes to put your thoughts into print. When I walk into a library these days, my brain melts as I consider the amount of human thought, effort, and life that is captured in all the books it contains.

With this in mind, I have a few important thank-yous to share:

First, thank you to my wife Joy, for being insane enough to take me on and stick with me, even when the fairy tale did not proceed as planned. You are my sounding board and helped me develop my ideas on our daily dog walks and our weekly ski trips. You tolerated me sitting writing on our holidays for years. I could not have written this book without your hours of advice and your ruthless editing. You are my everything. I adore you!

Thanks to my sons: Isaac, Joseph, Daniel, and Benjamin for inspiring me. You are all my heroes. Pick your parents carefully. Sorry, boys.

To my mum and dad, thank you for teaching me that the truth is out there. Thank you for loving me and always backing me. Thank you for introducing me to Jesus. Thank you to my sister, Sarah, and my brothers, Peter and Stephen, for your years of support and lovingly knocking the corners off me!

Thank you to my colleagues: All the doctors, nurses, medical office assistants, physios, students, and many other health care professionals who have taught me, worked with me, cried with me, laughed at me, and been there to listen to my latest ranting. Thank you for asking me so many questions and entertaining my answers. Thank you especially to Keith, Shauna, Janina, Dena, Bryce, Cinzia, Tim, Adam, Matt, Murray, Johan, Lu, Rob, Alex, Krish, Stephen, and Nav for taking the time to talk with me about my ideas.

Thank you to all my patients. I hope I have helped you. I always wish I had more time to spend with you because each of you is unique and valuable. Your journeys are fascinating. Each person I meet has something new to share and teach me. Thank you for hurting yourself in such inventive ways! I'm always impressed when you find new ways to injure yourselves.

Thank you to Britt Veenhuysen, my professional writer. You took my ramblings, processed them through the "Britt Machine" and out came a fantastic book. You are a genius. Contact Britt at www.brittanyveenhuysen.com if you need professional help with your book too.

Thank you, to my friend, Dean Winters for your witty cartoons. I'm hoping you will draw some more for me. He can draw for you too if you send him a request at echocreek@hotmail.com.

Thank you to my copy editor Tania Therien for your eagle-eyed review of my ~~grandma~~ grammar. She can fix your work too. Drop her a line at therientania@gmail.com.

Finally, thank you Tyler Massie for making the book look fantastic with your design and layout skills. Tyler can make you look good too at www.brandpsyche.ca.

Manufactured by Amazon.ca
Acheson, AB

10752052R00162